Prehospital Emergency Drugs

POCKET REFERENCE

KEVIN G. MADIGAN

Critical Care Flight Paramedic

reviewed by

Ronald D. Stewart, M.D.

The C. V. Mosby Company

St. Louis • Baltimore • Philadelphia • Toronto 1990

Editor Richard A. Weimer
Assistant editor Adrianne Cochran
Project manager Karen Edwards
Production Kathleen Teal
Cover art Alan Peak

Printed in the United States of America

The C.V. Mosby Company
11830 Westline Industrial Drive, St. Louis, Missouri 63146

Library of Congress Cataloging in Publication Data

Madigan, Kevin G.
Prehospital emergency drugs pocket reference / Kevin G. Madigan: reviewed by Ronald D. Stewart.
p. cm.
Includes bibliographical references.
ISBN 0-8016-3375-3
1. Medical emergencies—Handbooks, manuals, etc. 2. Drugs--Handbooks, manuals, etc. I. Stewart, Ronald D. II. Title.
[DNLM: 1. Drug Therapy—handbooks. 2. Emergencies—handbooks. 3. Emergency Medical Services—handbooks. WB 39M182p]
RC86.8.M325 1990
615'.7—dc20
DNLM/DLC
for Library of Congress

89-13702
CIP

C/PC/PC 9 8 7 6 5 4 3 2 1

Content Reviewers

Ronald D. Stewart, M.D., F.A.C.E.P., F.R.C.P.(C).
Director, Emergency Services, Sunnybrook Medical Centre,
Professor of Anesthesia, University of Toronto,
Toronto, Ontario, Canada

Brian P. Egier, M.D., F.R.C.P.(C).
Lecturer, Department of Anesthesia & Critical Care Medicine,
Sunnybrook Medical Centre, University of Toronto,
Toronto, Ontario, Canada

John F. Edmonds, M.B., B.S., F.R.C.P.(C).
Assistant Director, Department of Critical Care, Intensive Care Unit,
The Hospital for Sick Children,
Toronto, Ontario, Canada

Peter W. Skipper, M.B.B.S.
Associate Staff, Department of Critical Care, Intensive Care Unit,
The Hospital for Sick Children,
Toronto, Ontario, Canada

Don Stewart, B.A.Sc., M.D.
Emergency Physician, Base Hospital Medical Director,
Cambridge Memorial Hospital,
Cambridge, Ontario, Canada

Bruce Dewar, BSc, C.C.N.
Critical Care Nurse,
Sunnybrook Medical Centre / Bandage 1,
Toronto, Ontario, Canada

Charles Brault, M.I.C.P.
Mobile Intensive Care Paramedic,
New York City, New York

John A. Hubert, E.M.C.A., C.C.A.
Coordinator, Advanced Life Support Program, Sunnybrook Medical Centre,
Toronto, Ontario, Canada

Ahmed Coovadia
Blood Bank,
Charge Technologist, Sunnybrook Medical Centre,
Toronto, Ontario, Canada

Sheila Haddad
Blood Bank,
The Hospital for Sick Children,
Toronto, Ontario, Canada

Paramedic Consultants

Andy deBoer, C.C.F.P.
Critical Care Flight Paramedic, Sunnybrook Medical Centre / Bandage 1,
Toronto, Ontario, Canada

Colleen Rafton, C.C.F.P.
Critical Care Flight Paramedic, Sunnybrook Medical Centre / Bandage 1,
Toronto, Ontario, Canada

This book was inspired by the memory of two fine men, Gerald C. Madigan, my father, and Louis G. Madigan, my grandfather.

This pocket reference is dedicated to them, to present and future paramedics, and to those of you involved in the enhancement and proliferation of prehospital and interhospital medicine in Ontario, Canada.

Preface

During paramedic training, I found it difficult to find a drug book aimed at the needs of a paramedic. It did not take long to appreciate the complexity of a paramedic's job, especially the task of remembering drugs that we do not use often.

It became apparent that a practical and to-the-point pocket reference would be very useful in prehospital, interhospital, and emergency department settings. It might also provide a text for training.

This pocket reference is intended for paramedics and flight nurses. Content is aimed primarily at prehospital and interhospital emergency care and provides clinically relevant information. I hope that it will also prove valuable to emergency physicians, nurses, and ambulance personnel.

Prehospital Emergency Drugs Pocket Reference was not designed to be a comprehensive drug information source or to provide you with everything you need to know about pharmacologic agents. It was, however, designed to provide a strong knowledge base and rapid access to pertinent information in the prehospital emergency seting.

Kevin G. Madigan

Acknowledgments

Special recognition goes to Kathy Smuck, who typed the entire manuscript and assisted with the many drafts; to Grant Movold, for his computer expertise and continual assistance, and to Donna McKenna for her computer knowledge and of course for the use of her computer. Their patience and assistance through many manuscript drafts helped to produce this pocket reference.

Special thanks to Winnie Hobbs and the staff of Daniel Freeman Memorial Hospital Paramedic School in Inglewood, California, where I received paramedic training and certification; and to Dr. Peter Lane, Dr. Barry McLellan, Terri Burton, and Bryan Justice of Sunnybrook Medical Centre, Toronto, Ontario, where I received Critical Care Flight Paramedic training.

The many medical reviewers and editors, of course, deserve a great deal of credit. I would especially like to thank Dr. Ronald Stewart, known to many of us as a pioneering father of prehospital medicine (Dr. Stewart was instrumental in shaping the paramedic programs of Los Angeles and Pittsburgh), and Dr. Brian Egier for their very practical and meticulous review. Dr. John Edmonds and Dr. Peter Skippen were extremely helpful in their review of pediatric drug dosages.

I would also like to thank the many people whose encouragement kept me motivated throughout this project. Special thanks to Kathy, my family and friends, and to my co-workers, the flight paramedics, helicopter pilots, and engineers of Bandage 1.

Kevin G. Madigan

About the Author

Kevin G. Madigan is a critical care flight paramedic with Bandage 1-Helicopter 799 in Toronto, Ontario. He received paramedic training at Daniel Freeman Memorial Hospital Paramedic School in Los Angeles, California, and subsequently received critical care flight paramedic training at Sunnybrook Medical Centre, University of Toronto, Ontario, Canada.

Notice

This pocket reference contains widely accepted standards and recommendations from across the United States and Canada. The information presented conforms to current medical literature, to manufacturer product monographs, and to clinical practices of the general medical community at the time of publication. Nevertheless, this pocket reference should not be considered absolute or universal.

Standards, policies, and local protocols may differ between geographical areas and sometimes change rapidly, as research reveals new evidence. Although every effort has been made to ensure accuracy and completeness, the author, editors, medical advisors, consultants, and publisher disclaim liability for any discrepancies, incongruencies, undetected errors, omissions in content, or reader misunderstanding.

The author, editors, and advisors have produced this pocket reference on their own. No official support or endorsement from any hospital, university, college, association, service, or company is intended.

Contents

Section One

Adrenergic Receptors
Format of Drug Information
Symbols
Abbreviations

Adrenergic Receptor Cells of the Sympathetic Nervous System—A summary of alpha (α) and beta (β) effects

ALPHA$_1$ EFFECTS Peripheral vasoconstriction → ↑ BP

BETA$_1$ EFFECTS

1. (+) chronotropic → ↑ HR
2. (+) inotropic (↑ contractility) → improved output
3. (+) dromotropic (improves AV node conduction and shortens refractory period)
4. Improves automaticity
5. Increases myocardial irritability (excitability) → PVCs
6. Increases MVO_2 demand → angina; may increase infarct size

BETA$_2$ EFFECTS

1. Bronchodilation → improves vital capacity and tidal volume
2. Peripheral vasodilation → reduces afterload and preload

Predominant Alpha and Beta Effects on Organs

Smooth muscle location	Alpha (α) receptors	Beta (β) receptors
Cardiac	Few	β_1
Vascular	α_1	β_2
Bronchiolar	Few	β_2

DOPAMINERGIC EFFECTS Renal and mesenteric (splanchnic) vasodilation → improved renal and hepatic perfusion (see Dopamine)

FORMAT OF DRUG INFORMATION

Information generally pertains to emergency use.

GENERIC NAME(S) Trade Name(s)

TYPE: Therapeutic Classification

ACTIONS: Major mechanism(s) (how the drug exerts its therapeutic effects).

Onset	Peak	Duration
Elapsed time until the drug begins to exert its effects.	Elapsed time until the drug exerts its maximal effects.	Length of time the drug continues to exert its effects after administration is discontinued.

INDICATIONS & USES: Condition(s) for which the drug is recommended.

ADVERSE EFFECTS: Any side effect other than those that were therapeutically intended; usually undesirable, specific, and predictable; often a result of too rapid administration or too much of the drug. Boldface type generally indicates effects that are more common or life-threatening.

PRECAUTIONS: Condition(s) or relative contraindications that warrant cautious use of the drug; one should use caution in the presence of any adverse effect(s), or pregnancy, the very young, elderly, or debilitated.

INTERACTIONS: Presence of other drugs may have effects on the drug that you are giving. Drugs of a similar type may exert additive effects but are generally not included for the sake of brevity and simplicity.

CONTRA-INDICATIONS: Condition(s) where the drug should not be used (unless the benefits outweigh the risks). Drug hypersensitivity is an obvious precaution/contraindication but is not listed for every drug for the sake of brevity and simplicity.

GENERIC NAME(S)	Trade Name(s)

Note: Contraindications vary somewhat throughout the literature and among physicians.

PREPARATIONS: Amount/volume, container, and (concentration). Those most commonly carried on paramedic units.

DOSE: Amount commonly given for the condition, route, timing (slow IV → over 1-2 min), and repeat doses.
Drugs are *usually* diluted with NS or Sterile H_2O for Injection, and are mixed in either D_5W or NS for infusion, unless specified. Children younger than 18-24 months tend not to receive NS; other diluents include $D_{10}W$ or D_5 0.2 NS.

Note: Infant doses can be extremely complex and are generally beyond the scope of this pocket reference.

SPECIAL: Miscellaneous relevant or nice-to-know information.

IV INFUSION DOSAGE/FLOW RATE CHART:
Based on the standard microdrip calibration of 60 drops = 1.0 ml.
The diluent volume should be determined based on patient fluid requirements/restrictions.
The concentration may be changed by altering the amount of drug and volume of diluent solution. The flow rate should be adjusted depending on what concentration is used.

INTERHOSPITAL CONSIDERATIONS: This section is included primarily for emergency interhospital care personnel.

SYMBOLS

@	at
α	alpha
β	beta
pO_2	partial pressure of O_2
μ	micro
↑	increase (-s), (-ed), (-ing), elevated
↑ ↑	markedly increase (-s), (-ed), (-ing)
↓	decrease (-s), (-ed), (-ing)
↓ ↓	markedly decrease (-s), (-ed), (-ing)
(+)	positive, plus
(−)	negative, minus
±	plus/minus
↔	reversible reaction
→	leads (-ing) to, going to, implies
>	greater than
<	less than
≦	less than or equal to
=	equal(s)
≅	approximately equals
#	number, fracture
2°	second degree
∴	therefore

ABBREVIATIONS

a.c.	before meals
ACh	acetylcholine
admin.	administer, administration
amp.	ampule
amt.	amount
b.i.d.	2× daily
caps.	capsule
d.	daily
D/C, d/c	discontinue
g	gram, gauge
gr	grain
gtt(s)	macrodrop(s)
IM	intramuscular
inj.	injection
IO	intraosseous
IU	international unit
IV	intravenous
kg	kilogram
L	liter
MAX	maximum
mg	microgram
mEq	milliequivalent
min	minute(s), minimum
mg	milligram
ml	milliliter
mmol	millimole
mOsm	milliosmole
OD	overdose
p.c.	after meals
PO, po	by mouth
PR, pr	per rectum
prep.	preparation, prepare
p.r.n.	as required
Q, q	every
q.i.d.	4× daily
SC, SQ	subcutaneous
SL	sublingual
sol'n	solution
ss	one half
stat	at once
tab.	tablet
t.i.d.	3× daily
TKVO	to keep vein open
U, u	unit
µg	microgram
µgtt	microdrop
USP	United States Pharmacopeia
vol.	volume
Wt, wt	weight
y/o	year old
yr	year

Section Two

Drugs

AMINOPHYLLINE

TYPE: **Bronchodilator (Theophylline derivative)**

ACTIONS:
1. Bronchodilation & venodilation
2. Respiratory center & diaphragm stimulant
3. Mild diuretic
4. (+) chronotrope
5. (+) inotrope (in larger doses)

	Onset	Peak	Duration
IV	<15 min	<30 min	4½ hr

INDICATIONS & USES:
1. Bronchospasm (associated with asthma, chronic bronchitis, or emphysema)
2. Bronchospasm associated with pulmonary edema

ADVERSE EFFECTS:[1]

CVS
- □ **Tachycardia, palpitation, PVCs,** angina
- □ **Hypotension,** flushing, cerebral vasoconstriction

CNS
- □ **Dizziness,** drowsiness, nervousness, **anxiety,** headache, **tremor, seizure**

Other
- □ N/v, abdominal cramps, hematemesis, tinnitus

PRECAUTIONS:
1. Cardiac, hepatic, or renal insufficiency; AMI
2. Patients on a theophylline preparation[2]

INTERACTIONS:
1. β-blockers: may oppose effects
2. Barbiturates, Phenytoin, smoking: decreases theophylline levels

CONTRA-INDICATIONS:
1. Allergy to xanthine compounds (e.g., caffeine)
2. PVCs, tachycardia, arrhythmia

PREPARATIONS:
500 mg/10 ml ampule (50 mg/ml)
500 mg/20 ml ampule, preload (25 mg/ml)
250 mg/10 ml ampule, preload (25 mg/ml)

---

[1]Especially in hypoxic patients, from large doses, from rapid administration or from cardiac, renal, or hepatic insufficiency.
[2]Reduce dose (by ½) if patient has had a theophylline preparation within the past 6-24 hr.

DOSE:[3]		Draw bloods prior to administration (if possible)
	Adult	4-6 mg/kg in 50-250 ml, IV infusion @ $<$20 mg/min
	Child	5-7 mg/kg in 50-250 ml, IV infusion @ $<$20 mg/min
SPECIAL:		Therapeutic to toxic ratio is narrow
INTERHOSPITAL CONSIDERATIONS		
Dose:	**Adult**	Maintenance infusion 0.3-1 mg/kg/hr
	Child	Maintenance infusion 1 mg/kg/hr

[3]See footnote 2.

AMYL NITRITE

TYPE: **Coronary Vasodilator (Nitrite)**

ACTIONS:
1. Changes cyanide ion to a less harmful form
2. Reduces MVO_2 (via coronary vasodilation)

	Onset	Peak	Duration
Inhale	30 sec	1-2 min	3-20 min

INDICATIONS & USES: Cyanide poisoning[4]

ADVERSE EFFECTS:

CVS
- **Hypotension, reflex tachycardia,** palpitation, flushing, syncope

CNS
- **Transient headache,** transient dizziness, weakness, anxiety

Other
- N/v, allergic reaction
- Strong odor

PRECAUTIONS:
1. Cerebral hemorrhage, head injury
2. Vapors are highly flammable

INTERACTIONS: None significant

CONTRA-INDICATIONS: None when used for cyanide poisoning

PREPARATIONS: 0.3 ml/glass ampule (capsule)

DOSE:

Adult Place crushed capsule inside O_2 mask
Inhale vapor (1 crushed ampule) for 30-60 sec
Repeat q 5 min, until conscious

Child Same as adult

> **Note:** Deep breathing, head low posture, & movement of extremities may help relieve some adverse effects.

SPECIAL:
1. Has potential for tolerance & abuse (claimed to be an aphrodisiac)
2. Also known as "amy"

---

[4]Cyanide poisoning often produces a bitter almond breath odor.

TYPE: **Parasympatholytic-Vagal Blocker, Anticholinergic**

ACTIONS:
1. Blocks vagal effects resulting mostly in:
   a. (+) chronotropy
   b. (+) dromotropy
2. Anticholinergic (decreases bodily secretions)
3. Increases CNS stimulation
4. Some vasodilation

	Onset	Peak	Duration
IV	Immediate	1-4 min	2-6 hr

INDICATIONS & USES:
1. Hemodynamically significant bradycardia
2. Asystole
3. Organophosphate poisoning[5] (drug of choice)
4. Pre-intubation (especially in children)

ADVERSE EFFECTS:

CVS
- **Tachycardia, palpitation,** angina, PVCs, VF
- Possible hypotension

CNS
- **Headache, dizziness,** drowsiness, **anxiety**
- Confusion, hallucinations, delirium, coma

Other
- Anticholinergic effects:
  a. **Dry mouth/nose,** difficulty swallowing/talking
  b. **Pupil dilation, photophobia, blurred vision**
  c. Acute **urine retention**
- N/v, fever; flushed, hot, dry skin

PRECAUTIONS:
1. Hepatic or renal insufficiency; hypoxia or cyanosis
2. COPD (dries up secretions → mucous plugs)
3. Paradoxical bradycardia may occur if adult dose is <0.5 mg (child dose <0.1 mg), or if dose is given too slowly (usually lasts <2 min)

[5]Organophosphate poisoning generally causes increased body secretions.

ATROPINE

INTERACTIONS: Anticholinergics: may increase vagal blockade

CONTRA-INDICATIONS: Tachycardia

PREPARATIONS:
1 mg/10 ml preload (0.1 mg/ml)
0.5 mg/5 ml preload (0.1 mg/ml)
1 mg/1 ml ampule (1 mg/ml)

DOSE:

Adult ***Bradycardia:*** 0.5 mg rapid IV (or ETT)
Asystole: 1 mg rapid IV (or ETT)
Repeat q 5 min, p.r.n., MIN 0.5 mg, MAX 2 mg

Child ***Bradycardia/Asystole:***
0.02 mg/kg rapid IV (or ETT, IO)
Repeat q 5-20 min, p.r.n., MIN 0.1 mg, MAX 1 mg

Organophosphate Poisoning[6]:

Adult 2-4 mg rapid IV (or IM; 1 mg IV & 2 mg IM)
Repeat 2-4 mg rapid IV q 5-10 min, p.r.n.[7]

Child 0.05 mg/kg rapid IV (or IM)
Repeat q 5-10 min, p.r.n.[8]

SPECIAL:
1. May be reversed with Physostigmine (Antilirium)
2. 2 mg generally results in full vagal blockade

INTERHOSPITAL CONSIDERATIONS

Indications & Uses: In conjunction with Succinylcholine (to reduce salivation & potential for bradycardia)

---

[6]Patient should be well oxygenated to minimize risk of VF.
[7]To decrease secretions or until signs of full atropinization appear.
[8]See footnote 7.

BRETYLIUM

TYPE: **Antifibrillatory,[9] Antiarrhythmic (class III)**

ACTIONS:

1. Elevates the threshold for VF & may reduce energy required for successful defibrillation
2. Suppresses reentry arrhythmias
3. Initial sympathomimetic effects (≦ 20 min), followed by blockade (within 1-2 hr)
4. (+) inotrope
5. Transient (+) dromotrope

IV	Onset	Peak	Duration
VF	2-15 min	30 min-2 hr	2-6 hr
VT	20 min-6 hr	6-9 hr	up to 24 hr

INDICATIONS & USES:

1. Refractory VF, VT
2. Refractory PVCs

ADVERSE EFFECTS:

CVS
- □ Possible transient increased BP or HR
- □ **Hypotension, syncope, bradycardia**

CNS
- □ **Vertigo, dizziness**

Other
- □ Severe n/v (from rapid administration)

PRECAUTIONS:

1. Patient should be supine
2. Hepatic or renal insufficiency
3. May transiently exacerbate "Dig" toxicity
4. Prolonged hypotension post-resuscitation

INTERACTIONS:

1. Antihypertensives: potentiate hypotension
2. Sympathomimetics: potentiate pressor effects

CONTRA-INDICATIONS:

1. None for life-threatening arrhythmia
2. Any fixed cardiac output (e.g., Hx of aortic stenosis/pulmonary hypertension)

PREPARATIONS: 500 mg/10 ml ampule, preload (50 mg/ml)

[9] Appears to be more effective as an antifibrillatory agent.

BRETYLIUM

Bretylate
Bretylol

DOSE: **Adult** *VF:* 5 mg/kg rapid IV

> **Note:** Usually effective only if followed by defibrillation.

Repeat 10 mg/kg q 15-30 min p.r.n., MAX 30 mg/kg
IV infusion 1 g/250 ml @ 1-4 mg/min

VT: 5-10 mg/kg in 50 ml, IV infusion over 8-10 min
Repeat q1-2h p.r.n., MAX 30 mg/kg
or 1 g/250 ml @ 1-4 mg/min

Child Safety & efficacy not well established

> **Note:** *Cardiac arrest:* Use bolus therapy only. After resuscitation, consider infusion.
> *Recurrent arrhythmia or PVCs:* Repeat bolus & increase infusion rate by 1 mg/min.
> *Prevention:* Bolus & follow with infusion.

SPECIAL: VT does not respond as rapidly as does VF.

IV INFUSION DOSAGE/FLOW RATE CHART

For a **1 g/250 ml solution (4 mg/ml)**

Desired dose (mg/min)	Flow rate (ml/hr)
1	15
2	30
3	45
4	60

TYPE: **Calcium Salt (Electrolyte, Replenisher)**
Hypertonic Solution of Calcium & Chloride in Water

ACTIONS:
1. (+) inotrope
2. Enhances automaticity

	Onset	Peak	Duration
IV	Immediate		½-2 hr

INDICATIONS & USES:
1. Ca^{++} channel blocker OD
2. Hyperkalemic cardiac arrest
3. Adjunct therapy for toxins of insect bites/stings (especially black widow spider & scorpion)

ADVERSE EFFECTS:

CVS
- **Hypotension, bradycardia, arrhythmia, asystole, VF**
- May cause cerebral or coronary vasospasm

Other
- Chalky or metallic taste
- Warmth, pain, burning, or phlebitis extending from IV site; tingling; "heat waves"; sclerosis or thrombosis

PRECAUTIONS: Extravasation causes tissue necrosis

INTERACTIONS:
1. "Dig": potentiates effects → "Dig" toxicity
2. "Bicarb": precipitates, turns to "chalk"

CONTRA-INDICATIONS: "Dig" toxicity

PREPARATIONS: 1 g/10 ml preload, ampule (100 mg/ml) 10%

DOSE:

Adult 2-4 mg/kg slow IV @ <100 mg/min
Repeat q 10-20 min, p.r.n., MAX 1 g

Child 5-7 mg/kg slow IV over 5-10 min (or IO)
Repeat after 10-20 min, p.r.n., x1, MAX 300 mg

CALCIUM CHLORIDE

SPECIAL: Also known as $CaCl_2$.

INTERHOSPITAL CONSIDERATIONS

Indications & Uses:
1. Multiple rapid blood transfusions[10]
2. Hypocalcemia (e.g., inadequate cardiac output)
3. Hypermagnesemia

[10]Anticoagulants in banked blood bind to free Ca^{++}.

TYPE: **Adsorbent**

ACTIONS: Binds a wide variety of substances, inhibiting their GI absorption

	Onset	Peak	Duration
PO	Immediate	Immediate	Continual in GI tract

Note: Not absorbed, excreted in feces

INDICATIONS & USES: Practically all oral poisonings & ODs:
a. In conjunction with Ipecac
b. When emesis is contraindicated

ADVERSE EFFECTS: **Other**
- □ May indirectly induce n/v
- □ May clump in lower GI tract (→ constipation)[11]

PRECAUTIONS:
1. Does not absorb all drugs & toxic substances [12]
2. Decreased LOC (actual or potential)

INTERACTIONS: Ipecac: absorbed by "AC"

CONTRA-INDICATIONS: Corrosives, caustics, or petroleum distillates (relatively ineffective & may induce vomiting)

PREPARATIONS:
25 g (black powder)/125 ml bottle (200 mg/ml)
50 g (black powder)/250 ml bottle (200 mg/ml)

[11]Often followed with a cathartic (some include a cathartic).
[12]Does not adsorb cyanide. Relatively ineffective in adsorbing ethanol, methanol, alkalis, mineral acids, iron, lithium, magnesium, water insoluble compounds, most elemental compounds, & organophosphates.

DOSE: About 5-10× the amount of the poison (larger amounts if food is also present)

Adult 0.5-1 g/kg diluted to a 500 ml aqueous slurry, PO (or gastric tube), 10 min after Ipecac
Repeat 30 min after emesis is complete

Child 0.6-2 g/kg diluted 3× with H_2O, PO (or gastric tube), 10 min after Ipecac, give slowly
Repeat 0.5 g/kg, 30 min after emesis is complete

Note: Avoid use of milk, ice cream, sherbet, sweeteners, or juices to enhance palatability.[13]

SPECIAL:

1. Also known as "AC"
2. Relatively insoluble in H_2O
3. Will blacken feces
4. Must be stored in a closed container
5. Different Charcoal preparations may have varying adsorbing powers.

[13]Reduces adsorptive capacity.

TYPE: **Carbohydrate**
Hypertonic Solution of 50% Dextrose in Water

ACTIONS:
1. Immediate source of glucose & H_2O
2. Osmotic diuretic (transiently)

	Onset	Peak	Duration
IV	<1 min		depends on degree of hypoglycemia

INDICATIONS & USES: Any suspected hypoglycemia:
a. Altered LOC
b. Coma of unknown etiology[14]
c. Seizure of unknown etiology

ADVERSE EFFECTS: **Other** □ **Warmth, pain, burning, or phlebitis extending from IV site, sclerosis or thrombosis**

PRECAUTIONS:
1. Extravasation causes tissue necrosis
2. Alcoholics,[15] dehydration
3. Suspected intracranial hemorrhage, CVA

INTERACTIONS: None significant

CONTRA-INDICATIONS: None significant

PREPARATIONS:
25 g/50 ml preload ($D_{50}W$) (500 mg/ml)
12.5 g/50 ml preload ($D_{25}W$) (250 mg/ml)

DOSE: Draw bloods prior to administration (if possible).

Adult 12.5-25 g $D_{50}W$ slow IV
Repeat p.r.n., ×1

Child 0.5-1 g/kg $D_{25}W$ slow IV (or $D_{50}W$, diluted 1:1)
Repeat p.r.n., ×1

Note: Aspirate[16] occasionally to *ensure route patency*.

SPECIAL: Also known as $D_{50}W$

[14]Only if blood glucose levels are not immediately available.
[15]$D_{50}W$ may sometimes precipitate severe neurological symptoms (Wernicke's encephalopathy) in thiamine-deficient patients, which can be prevented with Thiamine (100 mg IV).
[16]Draw back on the barrel looking for blood return.

DIAZEPAM — Valium

TYPE: **Anticonvulsant, Sedative**

ACTIONS:
1. Suppresses (limits) spread of seizure activity & raises the seizure threshold (in the motor cortex)
2. Depresses the CNS, transient analgesia
3. Muscle relaxation

	Onset	Peak	Duration
IV	1-5 min	15 min	15 min-1 hr
IM	15-30 min	30-45 min	15 min-1 hr
PR	Rapid	15-30 min	15 min-1 hr

Note: Most rapid IV onset of all anticonvulsants

INDICATIONS & USES:
1. Initial Tx of seizures (drug of choice)
2. Sedation

ADVERSE EFFECTS:

CVS
- **Hypotension,**[17] reflex tachycardia

CNS
- **Respiratory depression/apnea,**[18] excessive CNS depression, drowsiness, ataxia, transient amnesia
- May paradoxically exacerbate seizure

Other
- **Warmth, pain, burning, or phlebitis** extending from IV site; may cause thrombosis
- N/v

PRECAUTIONS:
1. Already compromised respiratory status
2. Elderly (sensitive), children (unpredictable)
3. May precipitate if diluted

INTERACTIONS: CNS depressants: potentiate sedative effects

CONTRA-INDICATIONS: Hypoglycemic seizure (use Dextrose)

PREPARATIONS:
20 mg/2 ml ampule, preload (10 mg/ml)
10 mg/2 ml ampule, preload (5 mg/ml)

[17] Especially if administered too rapidly, to the elderly, or to patients with pulmonary disease. Be prepared to resuscitate.
[18] See footnote 17.

Valium — DIAZEPAM

DOSE:

Adult ***Seizures:*** 2-10 mg slow IV @ <5 mg/min
Repeat q 5-15 min, p.r.n., MAX ≅ 30 mg
Sedation: 2-5 mg slow IV @ <5 mg/min (or IM)
Repeat q 3-4 h p.r.n.

Child 0.2 mg/kg slow IV @ <1 mg/min (or PR, IO)
Repeat q 5-15 min, p.r.n., MAX ≅ 20 mg

> **Note:** Have resuscitation equipment readily available.

SPECIAL: Also a common prescription drug

DIAZOXIDE — Hyperstat

TYPE: **Antihypertensive**

ACTIONS: Arteriolar vasodilation

	Onset	Peak	Duration
IV	<5 min	<5 min	<12 hr

INDICATIONS & USES: Hypertensive crisis

ADVERSE EFFECTS:

CVS
- Severe persistent **hypotension,** bradycardia, flushing, syncope
- Reflex tachycardia, palpitation, angina, PVCs
- Na^+ & H_2O retention → CHF, edema

CNS
- **Headache,** dizziness, sweating

Other
- **N/v,** abdominal pain, tinnitus
- May cause warmth, pain, burning, or phlebitis extending from IV site

PRECAUTIONS:
1. Reduce BP slowly
2. Extravasation may cause tissue necrosis
3. Impaired organ perfusion (especially cerebral)
4. Cardiac, hepatic, or renal insufficiency
5. May arrest labor (from uterine relaxation)

INTERACTIONS: Anticoagulants: may potentiate effects

CONTRA-INDICATIONS:
1. Compensatory hypertension
2. Dissecting aneurysm
3. Allergy to thiazide derivatives

PREPARATIONS: 300 mg/20 ml ampule (15 mg/ml)

DOSE:

Adult 1-2 mg/kg rapid IV over <30 sec
Repeat q 5-15 min, p.r.n.

Child Same as adult

Note: A β-blocker should be available for reflex tachycardia.

SPECIAL: Often used with a diuretic to enhance the antihypertensive effect & reduce Na^+ retention

Gravol
Dramamine

DIMENHYDRINATE

More common in interhospital use

TYPE: **Antiemetic**

ACTIONS: Uncertain, probably affects neural pathways to inhibit n/v

	Onset	Peak	Duration
IV	Immediate	1-3 hr	3-6 hr
IM	20-30 min		3-6 hr
PO	15-30 min		3-6 hr

Note: Most effective when given prophylactically

INDICATIONS & USES:

1. Prevention/relief of n/v
2. Prevention/relief of motion sickness

ADVERSE EFFECTS:

CVS
- □ Hypotension, reflex tachycardia, palpitation

CNS
- □ CNS depression, **drowsiness,** dizziness, weakness, headache, anxiety, excitement, ataxia, seizure

Other
- □ Blurred vision; tinnitus; dry mouth, nose, & bronchi
- □ Warmth, pain, burning, or phlebitis extending from IV site (if undiluted)

PRECAUTIONS:

1. Seizure disorders
2. Asthmatics

INTERACTIONS: CNS depressants: potentiate depressant effects

CONTRA-INDICATIONS: None significant

PREPARATIONS:

50 mg/5 ml vial, ampule (10 mg/ml)
50 mg/1 ml ampule (50 mg/ml)
50 mg/2 ml vial (25 mg/ml)

DOSE:

Adult 12.5-25 mg (diluted) slow IV (or 50-100 mg IM, PO) or minibag
Repeat q4h, p.r.n.

Child Uncommon

SPECIAL: Also a common over-the-counter drug

DIPHENHYDRAMINE — Benadryl

TYPE: **Antihistamine**

ACTIONS:
1. Inhibits histamine release
2. CNS depressant
3. Anticholinergic, antiemetic

	Onset	Peak	Duration
IV	Immediate	1-4 hr	4-7 hr

INDICATIONS & USES:
1. Prevention/Tx of allergic reaction
2. Extrapyramidal reaction (e.g., phenothiazine OD)
3. Prevention/relief of motion sickness
4. Anxiety

ADVERSE EFFECTS:

CVS
- □ Hypotension, reflex tachycardia, palpitation

CNS
- □ CNS depression, **drowsiness,** dizziness, confusion
- □ Headache, anxiety, excitement (especially kids), ataxia, vertigo, seizure

Other
- □ **Dry mouth,** nose, & bronchi; blurred vision
- □ **N/v,** urine retention

PRECAUTIONS:
1. Asthmatics, COPD (may precipitate an attack)
2. Seizure disorders

INTERACTIONS: Atropine: potentiates anticholinergic effects

CONTRA-INDICATIONS: Asthmatic attack

PREPARATIONS:
50 mg/1 ml ampule, preload (50 mg/ml)
100 mg/10 ml vial (10 mg/ml)

DOSE:

Adult 10-50 mg slow IV (or deep IM, PO)
Repeat q4-6h, p.r.n.

Child 1-2 mg/kg slow IV (or deep IM, PO), MAX 50 mg
Repeat q4-6h, p.r.n.

SPECIAL:
1. Also a common over-the-counter drug
2. Supplied in some anaphylaxis kits (50 mg tablets)

More common in interhospital use

TYPE: **Sympathomimetic**

ACTIONS:
1. Direct β_1 effects → mostly:
   a. Potent (+) inotropy
   b. (+) dromotropy
2. Slight β_2 effects (vasodilation)

Note: Net hemodynamic effect of improved output & reduced peripheral resistance (comparable to a Dopamine-Nitroprusside combination)

	Onset	Peak	Duration
IV	<10 min	<10 min	<2-10 min

INDICATIONS & USES: Depressed myocardial function (low output); Cardiogenic shock, CHF (when indicated by central hemodynamic monitoring)

ADVERSE EFFECTS:

CVS □ May cause increased BP or HR, palpitation, angina, **PVCs,** tachycardia

CNS □ Headache, tremor

Other □ N/v

PRECAUTIONS: Signs of myocardial ischemia

INTERACTIONS:
1. β-blockers: may inhibit effects
2. Alkaline solutions: may inactivate

CONTRA-INDICATIONS:
1. Hypovolemia (replenish volume 1st)
2. Uncorrected tachycardia

PREPARATIONS: 250 mg (white powder)/20 ml vial
Reconstitute: With 10-20 ml NS or Sterile Water for Injection

More common in interhospital use

DOSE: **Adult** 500 mg/250 ml, IV infusion @ 0.5-2.5 μg/kg/min
Increase by 2 μg/kg/min, p.r.n.,[19] MAX 20 μg/kg/min

Child Same as adult
Increase by 1 μg/kg/min, p.r.n., MAX 25 μg/kg/min

SPECIAL:
1. Sometimes used with Dopamine or Nitroprusside
2. Less adverse cardiac effects than Dopamine

IV INFUSION DOSAGE/FLOW RATE CHART
For a **500 mg/250 ml** solution **(2 mg/ml)**

Desired dose (μg/kg/min)	Patient body weight (kg)								
	35	40	50	60	70	80	90	100	110
1.0	1	1	2	2	2	2	3	3	3
2.0	2	2	3	4	4	5	5	6	7
2.5	3	3	4	5	5	6	7	8	8
5.0	5	6	8	9	11	12	14	15	16
10.0	10	12	15	16	21	24	27	30	33
15.0	16	18	23	27	32	36	41	45	50
20.0	21	24	30	36	42	48	54	60	66

Flow rate (ml/hr)

Note: For a **1 mg/ml** concentration, multiply flow rate by 2.

[19]To improve LOC, BP (>90/60 mm Hg, children >70 mm Hg), urine output, & to avoid tachycardia or PVCs.

Revimine
Intropin

DOPAMINE

TYPE: **Sympathomimetic**

ACTIONS: Dose dependent. *Generally* predominant:
a. *Dopaminergic* effects from 0.5-5 μg/kg/min
b. β_1 effects from 5-10 μg/kg/min
c. α effects from 10^+ μg/kg/min

Note: There is some "overlap." β_1 effects are minimal beyond 20 μg/kg/min.

	Onset	Peak	Duration
IV	<5 min	<10 min	<10 min

INDICATIONS & USES:
1. Cardiogenic shock (drug of choice)
2. Other shock states with hemodynamically significant hypotension[20]
3. Acute renal failure, CHF

ADVERSE EFFECTS:
CVS
- **Tachycardia, palpitation,** angina, **PVCs**
- **Hypotension** (low dose), hypertension (high dose)

CNS
- Headache, tremor

Other
- Warmth, pain, burning, or phlebitis extending from IV site, **n/v**

PRECAUTIONS:
1. Extravasation causes tissue necrosis
2. Hypovolemia (should replenish volume 1st, but may be required *transiently*)
3. Signs of excessive vasoconstriction

INTERACTIONS: Alkaline solutions: may inactivate

CONTRA-INDICATIONS: Uncorrected tachyarrhythmia

PREPARATIONS: 200 mg/5 ml ampule, preload (40 mg/ml)
400 mg/5 ml vial (80 mg/ml)

[20]Decreased LOC, systolic BP <90 mmHg with hypoperfusion, or oliguria, *unresponsive to fluid replacement.*

DOPAMINE

Revimine
Intropin

DOSE: **Adult** 400 mg/250 ml, IV infusion @ 2-5 μg/kg/min
Increase by 2-5 μg/kg/min, p.r.n.,[21] MAX 50 μg/kg/min

Child Same as adult (or IO)
Increase by 1 μg/kg/min, p.r.n.,[22] MAX 25 μg/kg/min

SPECIAL: Per kg dose may be higher in children than in adults to achieve comparable effects

IV INFUSION DOSAGE/FLOW RATE CHART

For a **400 mg/250 ml** solution **(1,600 μg/ml)**

Desired dose (μg/kg/min)	Patient body weight (kg)								
	35	40	50	60	70	80	90	100	110
1.0	1	1	2	2	3	3	4	4	4
2.0	3	3	4	5	5	6	7	8	8
2.5	3	4	5	6	7	8	8	9	10
5.0	7	8	9	11	13	15	17	19	21
10.0	13	15	19	23	26	30	34	38	41
15.0	20	23	28	34	39	45	51	56	62
20.0	26	30	38	45	52	60	68	75	83

Flow rate (ml/hr)

Note: For an **800 μg/ml** concentration, multiply flow rate by 2.

[21]To improve LOC, BP (>90/60 mmHg, children >70 mmHg), urine output & to avoid tachycardia or PVCs.
[22]See footnote 21.

TYPE: **Sympathomimetic**

ACTIONS:
1. β_1 effects
2. β_2 effects
3. α effects[23] (higher doses)
4. Inhibits histamine release

	Onset	Peak	Duration
IV	<2 min	<5 min	5-10 min
SC	3-10 min	20 min	20-30 min
ETT	<1 min	<5 min	5-10 min

INDICATIONS & USES:
1. Cardiac arrest
2. Allergic reaction
3. Bronchoconstriction, bronchospasm

ADVERSE EFFECTS:

CVS
- **Tachycardia, palpitation,** angina, PVCs
- Hypertension (high doses)
- Hypotension (low doses)

CNS
- **Nervousness,** anxiety, headache, tremor

Other
- N/v, pupil dilation

PRECAUTIONS:
1. >35 yr of age (cardiovascular disease)
2. Hypovolemia (should replenish volume 1st, but may be required *transiently*)

INTERACTIONS:
1. β-blockers: may inhibit β-effects
2. Alkaline solutions: may inactivate

CONTRA-INDICATIONS: Uncorrected tachyarrhythmia

PREPARATIONS:
1:10,000 1 mg/10 ml preload (0.1 mg/ml)
1:1000 1 mg/1 ml ampule, preload (1.0 mg/ml)

[23] Improves organ perfusion pressure, which is its most beneficial effect during cardiac arrest.

DOSE:

Cardiac Arrest:

Adult 1:10,000 0.5-1.0 mg rapid IV (or ETT)
Repeat q 5 min, p.r.n.

Child 1:10,000 0.01 mg/kg rapid IV (or ETT, IO)
Repeat q 5 min, p.r.n.

Allergic/Asthmatic:

Adult 1:10,000 0.1 mg slow IV (or ETT)
Repeat q 3-5 min, p.r.n. MAX 0.5 mg
or 1:1000 0.1-0.5 mg SC
Repeat q 5-30 min, p.r.n., MAX ×3

Child 1:10,000 0.1 mg/kg slow IV (or ETT)
Repeat q 5-20 min, p.r.n.
or 1:1000 0.01 mg/kg SC, MAX 0.5 mg
Repeat q 5-30 min, p.r.n., MAX ×3

Stings/Bites:

Use 1:1000, 0.1-0.5 mg SC @ the site.
Contraindicated on fingers, toes, ears, nose, & genitalia

Note: The 1:1000 solution should not be given IV or ETT. It may be diluted with 9 ml NS to produce a 1:10,000 (1 mg/10 ml) solution.

SPECIAL:

1. Also known as "Epi"
2. Supplied in the anaphylaxis kit, 1:1000 solution, 1 mg/1 ml preload
3. New EpiPen auto-injector (0.5 mg/ml) 1:2000. Adult (0.3 mg/0.6 ml), child (0.15 mg/0.3 ml).

More common in interhospital use

TYPE: **Narcotic (Opiate) Analgesic**

ACTIONS:
1. Analgesia
2. Sedation, anesthesia

Note: Respiratory depressant effect may persist longer than analgesic effect

	Onset	Peak	Duration
IV	Immediate	3-15 min	30-90 min

Note: About 80× more potent, faster onset, and shorter duration than Morphine.

INDICATIONS & USES:
1. An alternative to paralyzation in patients with potential for seizures
2. Short-acting analgesia & sedation

ADVERSE EFFECTS:

CVS
- **Hypotension, bradycardia**

CNS
- **Respiratory depression/apnea, CNS depression**
- **Euphoria,** drowsiness, sedation, weakness
- Paradoxical CNS stimulation, nervousness, anxiety, headache, seizure, coma

Other
- N/v, **urine retention; muscle rigidity,** laryngospasm, bronchoconstriction
- May suppress cough or corneal reflex
- Pupil constriction, blurred vision

PRECAUTIONS:
1. When CNS status requires close monitoring
2. Pain of unknown etiology, multiple trauma
3. Hepatic or renal insufficiency
4. Seizure disorders

INTERACTIONS: CNS depressants, TCAs, MAOIs: potentiate effects

CONTRA-INDICATIONS: Presence of MAOIs within 14 days

More common in interhospital use

PREPARATIONS: 100 μg/2 ml ampule (50 μg/ml)
250 μg/5 ml ampule (50 μg/ml)

DOSE:

Adult 25-50 μg (diluted) slow IV
Repeat q 30-60 min, p.r.n.

Child 0.5-1 μg/kg (diluted) slow IV
Repeat q 30-60 min, p.r.n.

Note: Have a narcotic antagonist & resuscitation equipment readily available.

SPECIAL:

1. Commonly used in the OR as premedication for anesthesia
2. Has less emetic activity than other narcotics

TYPE: **Diuretic**

ACTIONS:

1. Vasodilation
2. Diuresis

IV	Onset	Peak	Duration
Vasodilation	<5-10 min	30 min	<2 hr
Diuresis	5-30 min	20-60 min	6 hr

INDICATIONS & USES:

1. Acute pulmonary edema, CHF
2. Hypertensive crisis

ADVERSE EFFECTS:[24]

CVS
- □ **Hypovolemia, hypotension,** arrhythmia

Other
- □ Excessive diuresis, **fluid/electrolyte imbalance, dehydration**
- □ Visual or auditory disturbances; vertigo
- □ N/v, abdominal pain

PRECAUTIONS:

1. Allergy to sulfas or thiazides
2. Cardiogenic shock, MI, renal insufficiency
3. Should be catheterized if transport >15 min

INTERACTIONS: None significant

CONTRA-INDICATIONS:

1. Anuria (except acute)
2. Hypokalemia[25]

PREPARATIONS:

20 mg/2 ml ampule, preload (10 mg/ml)
40 mg/4 ml ampule, preload (10 mg/ml)
100 mg/10 ml ampule, preload (10 mg/ml)

DOSE:[26]

Adult 20-40 mg slow IV (or IM)
Repeat q30 min, p.r.n., MAX 2 mg/kg

Child 0.5-1 mg/kg slow IV (or IM)
Repeat q30 min, p.r.n., MAX 2 mg/kg

[24]Mostly from high dose & long-term use; unlikely to present in the prehospital setting.
[25]Suspected in patients on chronic diuretic therapy with ECG showing prominent P-waves, diminished T-waves, present U-waves, muscle weakness, or cramps.
[26]May require larger doses in patients on diuretics or in renal failure.

FURОSEMIDE Lasix

SPECIAL:		Also a common prescription drug
INTERHOSPITAL CONSIDERATIONS		
Indications & Uses:		Acute renal failure
Dose:	**Adult**	IV infusion @ 4 mg/min

TYPE: **Pancreatic Hormone-Insulin Antagonist**

ACTIONS:
1. Indirectly raises blood glucose levels
2. Stimulates release of catecholamines → (+) inotropic & (+) chronotropic effects

	Onset	Peak	Duration
IM	5-20 min	<20 min	1-2 hr

INDICATIONS & USES:
1. Altered LOC where hypoglycemia is suspected & an IV route is not immediately available
2. β-blocker OD (see special)

ADVERSE EFFECTS:
CVS
- □ Possible tachycardia, hypertension

Other
- □ N/v
- □ Possible allergic reaction[27]

PRECAUTIONS: Hepatic or renal insufficiency

INTERACTIONS: None significant

CONTRA-INDICATIONS: Allergy to proteins

PREPARATIONS: 1 unit (mg) of white powder in one vial & 1 ml of fluid diluent in another vial (1 mg/ml)
Reconstitute: Only with diluent provided

DOSE:
Adult 0.5-1 mg IM (or SC)
Repeat in 20 min, p.r.n.

Child Same as adult, MAX 1 mg

Note: Administer IV glucose ASAP (if still unresponsive). Follow with oral carbohydrates when LOC improves.

SPECIAL: Sometimes used for β-blocker OD (adults 1 mg slow IV, repeat p.r.n.)

[27]Because it is a protein.

More common in interhospital use

TYPE: **Anticoagulant**

ACTIONS: Slows (prevents) blood clotting

	Onset	Peak	Duration
IV	Immediate	1-3 min	1 hr

INDICATIONS & USES:

1. Prevention of blood clot formation: post-MI, adjunctive (or post) thrombolytic therapy, pulmonary emboli, DVT, A-fib with emboli, frostbite, crush syndrome
2. Maintenance/patency for IV injection devices & catheters[28]
3. DIC (controversial)

ADVERSE EFFECTS:

CVS
- □ **Minor bleeding** to severe hemorrhage

Other
- □ May cause local irritation or pain at IV site
- □ Allergic reaction

PRECAUTIONS:

1. Patients on anticoagulants or thrombolytics
2. Cardiac, hepatic, or renal insufficiency; asthma
3. Avoid unnecessary vessel puncture; use small-gauge needle
4. Internal hemorrhage may be difficult to control; examine regularly for signs of bleeding

INTERACTIONS: Salicylates, some antibiotics, Quinidine: may increase risk of bleeding

CONTRA-INDICATIONS:

1. Risk of hemorrhage from any source
2. IM injection

---

[28]*Not* to be used for anticoagulant therapy.

More common in interhospital use

PREPARATIONS: 10,000 USP units/10 ml vial (1000 U/ml)
50,000 USP units/5 ml vial (10,000 U/ml)
Hepalean Lock Flush[29] 10 USP units/1 ml syringe, ampule (10 μ/ml)
Hepalean-Lok[30] 100 USP units/1 ml ampule (100 μ/ml)

DOSE:[31]

Adult 5000-10,000 U in 50 ml, slow IV over 15 min
Repeat q4h, p.r.n.
IV infusion 25,000 U/250 ml @ 1000-1500 U/hr

Child 50-100 U/kg in 50 ml, slow IV over 15 min
IV infusion @ 10-30 U/kg/hr

Flush 10-100 U, slow IV or a 2 U/ml solution @ 1.5-3 ml/hr

Note: Anticoagulation is adequate when PTT is 1½-2× control value (i.e., heparinized). Dosing is highly individualized.

SPECIAL: May be reversed with Protamine Sulphate
(1 mg/100μ of Heparin @ <50 mg/10min)

---

[29]See footnote 28.
[30]See footnote 28.
[31]Obtain coagulation times (PT, PTT) prior to administration.

HYDRALAZINE — Apresoline

More common in interhospital use

TYPE: **Antihypertensive**

ACTIONS: Arteriolar vasodilation

	Onset	Peak	Duration
IV	5-30 min	10-80 min	2-6 hr
IM	10-40 min	20-80 min	2-6 hr

INDICATIONS & USES:

1. Hypertension associated with renal failure, preeclampsia, eclampsia (drug of choice)
2. Hypertensive crisis

ADVERSE EFFECTS:

CVS
- **Reflex tachycardia, palpitation, angina**
- Hypotension, flushing

CNS
- **Headache,** dizziness, anxiety, paresthesia, tremor, sweating

Other
- **N/v,** muscle cramps

PRECAUTIONS:

1. Reduce BP slowly
2. Impaired organ perfusion (especially cerebral)
3. Cardiac, hepatic, or renal insufficiency

INTERACTIONS: Glucose solutions: may change color

CONTRA-INDICATIONS:

1. Compensatory hypertension
2. Dissecting aneurysm

PREPARATIONS: 20 mg/1 ml ampule (20 mg/ml)

DOSE:

Adult 10 mg slow IV (or IM)
Repeat q 10-15 min, p.r.n.
IV infusion 20 mg/250 ml NS or LR @ 5-20 mg/hr

Child 0.2 mg/kg slow IV
Repeat q 10-15 min, p.r.n.

Note: A β-blocker should be available for reflex tachycardia.

SPECIAL: Also a common prescription drug

TYPE: **Emetic**

ACTIONS: Induces vomiting of gastric contents

	Onset	Peak	Duration
PO	5-35 min	20-35 min	12-80 min

INDICATIONS & USES: Acute oral drug or toxin OD in alert patients[32] (drug & method of choice)

ADVERSE EFFECTS: **Other** □ Prolonged vomiting from OD

PRECAUTIONS:

1. Maintain & protect the airway
2. Decreased LOC (actual or potential)
3. Emesis may precipitate convulsions
4. Retching causes increased vagal tone

INTERACTIONS: Activated Charcoal: adsorbs Ipecac

CONTRA-INDICATIONS:[33]

1. Caustics, corrosives, petroleum distillates
2. Any patients who cannot protect their airway
3. Absent gag reflex[34]
4. Unknown ingestion
5. $<$9 mo of age

PREPARATIONS:

30 ml vial
15 ml vial

DOSE:

Adult 30-60 ml PO with 500 ml tap H_2O
Child 15 ml PO with 200-400 ml tap H_2O

Note: If ineffective after 20-35 min, repeat ×1. If still ineffective, lavage (or Activated Charcoal).
Note: Emesis will not remove all ingested toxin. Save an emesis sample for lab evaluation. Follow with Activated Charcoal.

SPECIAL:

1. Also a common over-the-counter drug
2. Usually effective in antiemetic OD
3. Milk & carbonated drinks may delay emesis

[32] Patients in control of their airway & who have an intact gag reflex.
[33] Contact poison control center (if uncertain). Activated Charcoal is sometimes used when emesis is contraindicated.
[34] Patients can be conscious & not have a gag reflex.

ISOPROTERENOL — Isuprel

TYPE: **Sympathomimetic**

ACTIONS: Pure β-adrenergic stimulation:
a. β_1 effects
b. β_2 effects

	Onset	Peak	Duration
IV	Immediate	2 min	<8 min

INDICATIONS & USES: Temporary[35] control of hemodynamically significant bradycardia (refractory to Atropine)

ADVERSE EFFECTS:

CVS
- □ **Tachycardia, palpitation, PVCs, angina,** may extend infarct size, VT, VF
- □ Hypotension, flushing

CNS
- □ **Headache,** tremor, weakness, dizziness, anxiety, nervousness, sweating

Other
- □ N/v, pulmonary congestion

PRECAUTIONS:
1. Hepatic or renal insufficiency
2. D/c if signs of ischemia worsen
3. "Dig" toxicity or hypokalemia (exacerbates arrhythmia)

INTERACTIONS:
1. Alkaline solutions: may inactivate
2. β-blockers: inhibit effects

CONTRA-INDICATIONS:
1. Cardiac arrest[36]
2. Hypotension (use fluids or vasopressors)

PREPARATIONS: 1 mg/5 ml ampule, preload (0.2 mg/ml)
2 mg/10 ml preload (0.2 mg/ml)

---

[35] Until a pacemaker is available. Major benefit is when primary need is chronotropic support.
[36] It is now believed that α-effects may be of more benefit.

DOSE:

Adult 1 mg/500 ml, IV infusion @ 2 μg/min
Increase by 1-2 μg/min, p.r.n.,[37] MAX 10 μg/min

Child 1 mg/500 ml, IV infusion @ 0.1 μg/kg/min
Increase by 0.1 μg/kg/min, p.r.n., MAX 1.0 μg/kg/min

SPECIAL: Also used post-resuscitation until pacing is available

IV INFUSION DOSAGE/FLOW RATE CHART
For a **1 mg/500 ml** solution **(2 μg/ml)**

Desired dose (μg/min)	Flow rate (ml/hr)
1	30
2	60
3	90
4	120
5	150
10	300

Note: For a **4 μg/ml** concentration, divide flow rate by 2.

[37]To a HR of ≅ 60/min, BP of >90-100 mmHg systolic & to avoid angina, tachycardia, or PVCs.

ISOXSUPRINE Vasodilan

More common in interhospital use

TYPE: **Uterine Myovascular Relaxant (Vasodilator)**

ACTIONS:
1. Inhibits uterine contraction
2. β-stimulation

	Onset	Peak	Duration
IV	15 min-10 hr		5-10 min

INDICATIONS & USES: Premature labor[38] (to postpone premature birth)

ADVERSE EFFECTS:

CVS
- □ **Hypotension, tachycardia, palpitation**
- □ Maternal pulmonary edema, ARDS
- □ Fetal hypotension or tachycardia

CNS
- □ Dizziness, anxiety, tremor, weakness

Other
- □ Severe **n/v,** abdominal pain, rash

PRECAUTIONS:
1. Should have a (+) diagnosis of premature labor
2. D/c in the absence of a prompt response

INTERACTIONS: None significant

CONTRA-INDICATIONS:
1. When pregnancy continuation jeopardizes the mother or fetus
2. Hemorrhage
3. Severe preeclampsia or eclampsia

PREPARATIONS: 40 mg/8 ml ampule (5 mg/ml)

[38]Suitable patients: >20 wk gestation, intact amniotic membranes, cervical dilation <4 cm, & effacement <80%.

More common in interhospital use

DOSE: **Adult** 40 mg/250 ml, IV infusion @ 0.2 mg/min
Increase (after 15 min) by 0.1-0.2 mg/min, p.r.n., MAX 1 mg/min
Titrate to:
a. Inhibit contractions
b. A HR of <120/min, BP of >90/50 mmHg
c. A FHR of <160/min

Note: After 3 hr, reduce by 30% for a minimum 24 hr maintenance.

SPECIAL: Some prefer Ritodrine (Yutopar), which may have fewer adverse effects

TYPE: **Antiarrhythmic (class Ib), Local Anesthetic**

ACTIONS:
1. Suppresses PVCs
2. Suppresses reentry arrhythmias
3. Elevates the threshold for VF
4. Local anesthetic (suppresses cough & gag reflex)

	Onset	Peak	Duration
IV	<3 min	2-7 min	8-20 min
ETT	1-2 min	<5 min	10-20 min
Aerosol	<2 min	<5 min	10-20 min

INDICATIONS & USES:
1. Drug of choice for the following:
   a. PVCs, VT, VF
   b. Prophylactically post-PVC, VT, or VF conversion
   c. Prophylactically in suspected AMI
2. Facilitates ETT insertion (aerosol, jelly) in the conscious patient
3. Pre-intubation in head injuries[38a]

ADVERSE EFFECTS:

CVS
- □ Possible hypotension, bradycardia, conduction disturbances

CNS[39]
- □ **CNS depression, drowsiness, dizziness,** respiratory depression, slurred speech
- □ **Confusion,** excitement, **anxiety**
- □ **Tremor,** paresthesia/numbness/tingling, **seizure**

Other
- □ N/v, **visual or auditory disturbances**

PRECAUTIONS: *See footnote 39.*

INTERACTIONS: β-blockers, Dopamine: may precipitate toxicity

CONTRA-INDICATIONS: 3° AV blocks, "rate-related PVCs," bradycardia, idioventricular rhythms

---

[38a]Minimizes rise in ICP associated with intubation.

[39]Especially in CHF, AMI, hypoperfusion states, hypoxia, hepatic or renal insufficiency, & the elderly (especially >70 yr old) or debilitated (reduce dose by ½).

PREPARATIONS:
100 mg/5 ml preload (20 mg/ml) 2%
100 mg/10 ml preload (10 mg/ml) 1%
1 g/250 ml D_5W premix bag (4 mg/ml) 0.4%
1 g/5 ml preload (200 mg/ml) 20%
10 mg/metered dose aerosol spray
30 ml tube of jelly (20 mg/ml) 2%

DOSE:

Adult 1 mg/kg slow IV over >2 min (or ETT)
Repeat 0.5 mg/kg q 8-10 min, p.r.n., MAX 3 mg/kg
IV infusion 1 g/250 ml @ 2-4 mg/min

Note: For pre-intubation (head injuries), 1.5 mg/kg slow IV; wait @ least 90 sec. before instrumentation.

Child 1 mg/kg slow IV over >2 min (or ETT, IO)
Repeat q 5 min, p.r.n., MAX 3 mg/kg
IV infusion 120 mg/100 ml @ 10-50 μg/kg/min

Note: *Cardiac arrest:* Use bolus therapy only. After resuscitation, consider infusion.
Recurrent arrhythmia or PVCs: Repeat bolus & increase infusion rate by 1 mg/min.
Prevention: Bolus & follow with infusion.

Aerosol 6-10 sprays, hypopharynx (& nares) MAX 20 sprays

SPECIAL:
Also a new prescription drug, LidoPen auto-injector (200-400 mg IM, deltoid or thigh)

IV INFUSION DOSAGE/FLOW RATE CHART
For a **1 g/250 ml** solution **(4 mg/ml)**

Desired dose (mg/min)	Flow rate (ml/hr)
1	15
2	30
3	45
4	60

MANNITOL Osmitrol

More common in interhospital use

TYPE: **Osmotic Diuretic**
Hypertonic Solution of Mannitol in Water

ACTIONS:
1. Decreases cerebral edema & elevated ICP
2. Transiently increases intravascular volume
3. Promotes diuresis

IV	Onset	Peak	Duration
Reduces ICP Diuresis	15 min 1-3 hr	60-90 min <3 hr	3-8 hr 4-6 hr

INDICATIONS & USES:
1. Raised ICP or cerebral edema[40] (drug of choice)
2. Acute renal failure

ADVERSE EFFECTS:

CVS
- **Transient volume overload, pulmonary edema/CHF,** tachycardia, hypertension, angina
- Hypotension (from excessive diuresis)

CNS
- Headache, dizziness, tremor, seizure

Other
- **Electrolyte imbalance, cellular dehydration, H_2O intoxication,** acidosis
- N/v, blurred vision, fever, chills
- May cause warmth, pain, or phlebitis extending from IV site

PRECAUTIONS:
1. There should be a (+) diagnosis of raised ICP[41]
2. Catheterize & monitor urine output
3. Extravasation causes tissue necrosis
4. Hypotension (replenish fluids & "lytes" 1st)
5. Crystallized solution[42]

---

[40]Consult with neurosurgeon or trauma center is advised. There should be clinical evidence of rising ICP or a space-occupying lesion with shift (deteriorating neurological signs, lateralizing signs).
[41]See footnote 40.
[42]Rewarming to 70°C (heater or immersion) will redissolve crystals. *Cool to body temperature before use.*

More common in interhospital use

INTERACTIONS: None significant

CONTRA-INDICATIONS:
1. Severe hypotension, dehydration, or hyponatremia
2. Established anuria, pulmonary edema/CHF
3. Suspected ICH

PREPARATIONS: 100 g/500 ml premix bag (200 mg/ml) 20%

DOSE:

> **Note:** Should be in-line filtered
> **For elevated ICP:** Should at least be intubated & hyperventilated

Adult 0.25-2 g/kg, IV infusion over 15 min
Repeat after 30 min, if no effect

Child 0.2-0.5 g/kg, IV infusion over 30-60 min
Repeat after 30 min, if no effect

> **Note:** With an expanding intracranial lesion, the duration of action may be relatively short. Subsequent doses are progressively less effective.

SPECIAL: Effectiveness depends on large doses & an intact blood-brain barrier

MEPERIDINE
PETHIDINE — Demerol

TYPE: **Narcotic (Opiate) Analgesic**

ACTIONS:
1. Analgesia
2. Sedation

	Onset	Peak	Duration
IV	<1 min	20-25 min	2-4 hr
IM	10 min	30-60 min	2-4 hr

> **Note:** About 1/10 as potent as Morphine.

INDICATIONS & USES:
1. Moderate-severe pain
2. Anxiety, apprehension

ADVERSE EFFECTS:

CVS
- □ **Hypotension,** bradycardia, flushing

CNS
- □ **Respiratory depression/apnea, CNS depression**
- □ **Euphoria,** drowsiness, dizziness, weakness
- □ Paradoxical CNS stimulation, nervousness, anxiety, headache, seizure, coma

Other
- □ May suppress cough or corneal reflex
- □ **N/v, urine retention,** may dilate pupils

PRECAUTIONS:
1. When CNS status requires close monitoring
2. Pain of unknown etiology, multiple trauma
3. Hepatic or renal insufficiency
4. Seizure disorders

INTERACTIONS:
1. MAOIs, barbiturates: increased CNS excitation or depression (can be fatal)
2. CNS depressants, TCAs: potentiate effects
3. Phenytoin: decreases effects

CONTRA-INDICATIONS: Presence of MAOIs within 14 days

Demerol — MEPERIDINE / PETHIDINE

PREPARATIONS: 50 mg/1 ml ampule, tubex (50 mg/ml)
100 mg/1 ml ampule, tubex (100 mg/ml)

DOSE:

Adult 50-100 mg (diluted) slow IV @ <25 mg/min (or IM, SC)
Repeat q2-4h, p.r.n.

Child 1 mg/kg (diluted) slow IV @ <25 mg/min (or IM, SC)
Repeat q2-4h, p.r.n.

> **Note:** Have a narcotic antagonist & resuscitation equipment readily available.

SPECIAL: Commonly given with an antiemetic such as Dimenhydrinate

MORPHINE

TYPE: **Narcotic (Opiate) Analgesic**

ACTIONS:

1. Analgesia
2. Vasodilation → reduced MVO_2
3. Sedation

	Onset	Peak	Duration
IV	Immediate	20 min	2-7 hr
IM	$<$10 min	$<$30-60 min	$>$2-7 hr

INDICATIONS & USES:

1. Ischemic chest pain (drug of choice if unrelieved by "Nitro")
2. Severe pain (drug of choice)
3. Acute cardiogenic pulmonary edema
4. Anxiety, apprehension

ADVERSE EFFECTS:

CVS
- □ **Hypotension,** bradycardia, flushing

CNS
- □ **Respiratory depression/apnea, CNS depression**
- □ **Euphoria,** drowsiness, dizziness, weakness
- □ Paradoxical CNS stimulation, nervousness, anxiety, headache, seizure, coma

Other
- □ May suppress cough or corneal reflex
- □ **N/v, urine retention,** pupil constriction

PRECAUTIONS:

1. When CNS status requires close monitoring
2. Pain of unknown etiology, multiple trauma
3. Hepatic or renal insufficiency
4. Seizure disorders

INTERACTIONS: CNS depressants, TCAs, MAOIs: potentiate effects

CONTRA-INDICATIONS:

1. Presence of MAOIs within 14 days

PREPARATIONS: 2 mg/1 ml ampule (2 mg/ml)
10 mg/1 ml ampule, tubex (10 mg/ml)
10 mg/10 ml preload (1 mg/ml)

DOSE: **Adult** 2-5 mg (diluted) slow IV @ <1 mg/min (or IM, SC)
Repeat q 5-30 min, p.r.n., usual MAX 20 mg

Child 0.1-0.2 mg/kg (diluted) slow IV over 5 min (or IM, SC)
Repeat q2h, p.r.n.

Note: Have a narcotic antagonist & resuscitation equipment readily available.

SPECIAL: Also known as "Morph," "MS," "MSO_4"

NALBUPHINE — Nubain

TYPE: **Narcotic (Opiate) Analgesic**[43]

ACTIONS:
1. Analgesia
2. Sedation

	Onset	Peak	Duration
IV	2-3 min	20 min	3-6 hr

Note: About as potent as Morphine.

INDICATIONS & USES:
1. Moderate-severe pain
2. Anxiety, apprehension

ADVERSE EFFECTS:

CVS
- □ Hypotension, bradycardia, flushing

CNS
- □ **Respiratory depression/apnea, CNS depression**
- □ Euphoria, drowsiness, dizziness
- □ Paradoxical CNS stimulation, hallucinations, nervousness, anxiety, headache, hostility

Other
- □ **N/v,** blurred vision, abdominal cramps

PRECAUTIONS:
1. When CNS status requires close monitoring
2. Pain of unknown etiology, multiple trauma
3. Hepatic or renal insufficiency; MI
4. Seizure disorders

INTERACTIONS: CNS depressants: potentiate effects

CONTRA-INDICATIONS: Emotional instability

PREPARATIONS:
10 mg/1 ml ampule (10 mg/ml)
20 mg/1 ml ampule (20 mg/ml)

[43] Acts as an analgesic when no opiates are on board (may also reverse effects of opiates).

DOSE:

Adult 2-5 mg (diluted) slow IV (or IM, SC)
Repeat q3-6h, p.r.n., usual MAX 20 mg

Child Safety & efficacy not well established

Note: Have a narcotic antagonist & resuscitation equipment readily available.

SPECIAL: Has weak narcotic antagonist effects[44] (similar to Naloxone) & may precipitate withdrawal syndrome in narcotic-dependent persons

---

[44]See footnote 43.

NALOXONE Narcan

TYPE: **Narcotic (Opiate) Antagonist**

ACTIONS: Reverses most effects of nearly all narcotic & narcotic-like substances (may not reverse hypotension)

	Onset	Peak	Duration
IV	<2 min	<2 min	20 min-2 hr
IM	2-10 min	2-10 min	20 min-2 hr
ETT	2-10 min	2-10 min	20 min-2 hr

INDICATIONS & USES: Drug of choice:
1. Narcotic-induced respiratory depression
2. Decreased LOC or coma of unknown etiology

ADVERSE EFFECTS:
CVS □ Possible hypertension, tachycardia
Other □ N/v, may prolong clotting times

PRECAUTIONS:
1. May induce acute narcotic withdrawal syndrome in narcotic-dependent persons (including neonates of narcotic-dependent mothers)
2. Will not reverse nonopiate-induced respiratory depression

INTERACTIONS: None significant

CONTRA-INDICATIONS: None significant

PREPARATIONS:
0.4 mg/1 ml ampule, preload (0.4 mg/ml)
1 mg/1 ml ampule, preload (1 mg/ml)
2 mg/2 ml ampule, preload (1 mg/ml)
0.04 mg/2 ml ampule (0.02 mg/ml) neonatal

DOSE:

Adult 0.1-2 mg slow IV (or ETT, IM)
Repeat q 5 min, p.r.n.[45]
Usually effective by 10 mg (but may require more)

Child 0.01 mg/kg slow IV (or ETT, IM)
Repeat q 5 min, p.r.n.[46]
Usually effective after a total of 0.1 mg/kg

Note: May require additional doses if narcotic effects recur (since duration is shorter than that of most narcotics).

SPECIAL:

1. May reverse ETOH-induced coma
2. May improve circulation in refractory shock

[45]Some prefer to improve respirations & BP but not to wake the patient in out-of-hospital care (there is a risk of aspiration)
[46]See footnote 45.

NIFEDIPINE

Adalat
Procardia

TYPE: **Calcium (slow) Channel Blocker**
Antianginal, Antiarrhythmic (class IV)

ACTIONS: Blocks entry of Ca^{++} into cells (especially cardiac & vascular smooth muscle) →:
a. Vasodilation (including coronary)
b. (−) inotropec.
c. Relaxes & inhibits coronary artery spasm

	Onset	Peak	Duration
SL	1-5 min	20-30 min	2-5 hr
PO	5-20 min	1-2 hr	2-5 hr

INDICATIONS & USES:
1. Hypertensive crisis
2. Angina
3. Pulmonary edema (investigational)

ADVERSE EFFECTS:

CVS
- □ Hypotension, **reflex tachycardia,** palpitation
- □ **Flushing,** peripheral edema
- □ May exacerbate angina or CHF

CNS
- □ **Headache, dizziness,** nervousness, weakness

Other
- □ **N/v, heartburn,** cramps, nasal congestion, dyspnea

PRECAUTIONS:
1. Reduce BP slowly
2. Impaired organ perfusion (especially cerebral)

INTERACTIONS: β-blockers: may potentiate effects → heart failure

CONTRA-INDICATIONS:
1. Compensatory hypertension
2. Dissecting aneurysm

PREPARATIONS: 5-10 mg liquid-filled capsules

Adalat
Procardia

NIFEDIPINE

DOSE:

Adult 5-10 mg SL
Repeat q 30-60 min, p.r.n.

Child Not well established

Note: Puncture end of capsule with a needle & squeeze, or bite & chew.

Note: A β-blocker should be available for reflex tachycardia.

SPECIAL: Also a common prescription drug (capsule contains thick viscous fluid)

NITROGLYCERIN — Various Trade Names

TYPE: **Vasodilator**

ACTIONS:

1. Vasodilation (especially coronary) → reduced MVO_2 & improved output
2. Redistribution of coronary flow (to ischemic zones)
3. Relieves coronary vasospasm

	Onset	Peak	Duration
SL tablet	1-3 min	5-10 min	20-30 min
SL aerosol	<2 min	5-10 min	<30 min

Note: Antianginal onset precedes hemodynamic onset.

INDICATIONS & USES:

1. Ischemic chest pain, AMI (drug of choice)
2. CHF, pulmonary edema
3. Dilates veins for IV initiation (topical)

ADVERSE EFFECTS:

CVS
- **Hypotension,** bradycardia, paradoxical angina, **reflex tachycardia, palpitation**
- Possible reperfusion arrhythmias
- **Flushing,** feeling of warmth

CNS
- Transient **headache, dizziness,** weakness, anxiety

Other
- N/v, may cause SL burning sensation

PRECAUTIONS: Impaired organ perfusion (especially cerebral)

INTERACTIONS: ETOH: may potentiate hypotension

CONTRA-INDICATIONS:

1. Suspected tamponade or pericarditis
2. Uncorrected hypovolemia

PREPARATIONS:
0.3, 0.4, 0.6 mg tablets (100/bottle)
0.4 mg/metered dose aerosol spray

DOSE:

Adult Tablet 0.3-0.4 mg SL
Aerosol 1-2 sprays SL (or translingual)
Repeat q 5 min, p.r.n., MAX ×2

Child Safety & efficacy not established

SPECIAL:

1. Also known as "Nitro," "NTG," & "GTN"
2. Also a common prescription drug

INTERHOSPITAL CONSIDERATIONS

Actions:

	Onset	Peak	Duration
IV	<2 min	<5 min	<9 min

Indications & Uses:
1. Unstable angina (usually post-MI)
2. CHF (drug of choice)
3. Poor output children post cardiac surgery

Preparations: 50 mg/10 ml ampule (5 mg/ml)

Dose:

Adult 50 μg IV bolus
50 mg/250 ml glass bottle, IV infusion @ 5 μg/min
Increase by 5-10 μg/min q 5-10 min, p.r.n.
Usually effective by 50-200 μg/min

Child 50 mg/250 ml glass bottle, IV infusion @ 0.5-5 μg/kg/min
Increase by 1 μg/kg/min, p.r.n., MAX 10 μg/kg/min

Note: Standard tubing may absorb "Nitro" (up to 80%), as do many plastics & filters. Special tubing is available that minimizes absorption.

IV INFUSION DOSAGE/FLOW RATE CHART

	Dilution/concentration		
Desired dose (μg/min)	**25 mg/250 ml (100 μg/ml)**	**50 mg/250 ml (200 μg/ml)**	**100 mg/250 ml (400 μg/ml)**
5	3	2	1
10	6	3	2
20	12	6	3
30	18	9	5
40	24	12	6
50	30	15	8
100	60	30	15

Flow rate (ml/hr)

NITROPRUSSIDE — Nipride

More common in interhospital use

TYPE: **Antihypertensive**

ACTIONS:
1. Vasodilation → reduced MVO_2
2. Improves cardiac output

	Onset	Peak	Duration
IV	<1 min	1-5 min	1-10 min

INDICATIONS & USES:
1. Acute hypertensive crisis
2. CHF,[47] cardiogenic shock[48] (when indicated by central hemodynamic monitoring)

ADVERSE EFFECTS:

CVS[49]
- □ **Hypotension,** reflex tachycardia, palpitation, angina

CNS[50]
- □ CNS depression

Other
- □ Thiocyanate toxicity[51]
- □ May cause warmth, pain, burning, or phlebitis extending from IV site

PRECAUTIONS:
1. Reduce BP slowly
2. Impaired organ perfusion (especially cerebral)
3. Hepatic or renal insufficiency
4. Extravasation causes tissue necrosis

INTERACTIONS: Almost all drugs & solutions: incompatible

CONTRA-INDICATIONS:
1. Compensatory hypertension
2. Dissecting aneurysm

PREPARATIONS: 50 mg (powder)/15 ml vial
Reconstitute: With 2-3 ml D_5W *only.*
Normally has a faint brownish tint.

---

[47]Combined Tx with Dopamine often is more effective than either drug alone.
[48]See footnote 47.
[49]Usually only from too rapid BP reduction.
[50]See footnote 49.
[51]Nitroprusside is rapidly metabolized to thiocyanate. Toxicity will occur from rapid administration (>15 μg/kg/min) or from prolonged high-dose infusion.

More common in interhospital use

DOSE: **Adult** 50 mg/250 ml D_5W *only* (protect from light)
IV infusion @ 0.5 μg/kg/min
Increase by 0.2 μg/kg/min q 5 min, p.r.n.
Average 3 μg/kg/min, MAX 10 μg/kg/min[52]

Child Same as adult

Note: A β-blocker should be available for reflex tachycardia.

SPECIAL: Amyl Nitrite may reverse some OD effects

IV INFUSION DOSAGE/FLOW RATE CHART
For a **50 mg/250 ml** solution **(200 μg/ml)**

Desired dose (μg/kg/min)	Patient body weight (kg)								
	35	40	50	60	70	80	90	100	110
0.1	1	1	2	2	2	2	3	3	3
0.2	2	2	3	4	4	5	5	6	7
0.5	5	6	8	9	11	12	14	15	17
1	11	12	15	18	21	24	27	30	33
2	21	24	30	36	42	48	54	60	66
3	32	36	45	54	63	72	81	90	99
4	42	48	60	72	84	96	108	120	132
5	53	60	75	90	105	120	135	150	165
6	63	72	90	108	126	144	162	180	198
7	74	84	105	126	147	168	189	210	231
8	84	96	120	144	168	192	216	240	264

Flow rate (ml/hr)

Note: For a **400 μg/ml** concentration, divide flow rate by 2.

[52] If BP is not reduced in 10 min, d/c the infusion.

NITROUS OXIDE/OXYGEN

Entonox
Nitronox

TYPE: **Gaseous Analgesic**

ACTIONS:
1. Analgesia
2. Sedation

	Onset	Peak	Duration
Inhale	2-5 min	2-5 min	2-5 min

Note: Eliminated unchanged via the lungs in 2-5 min.

INDICATIONS & USES:
1. Temporary relief/prevention of pain from any source (provided no contraindications exist)
2. Conscious sedation (anxiety, apprehension)

ADVERSE EFFECTS:

CNS
- □ **Drowsiness, dizziness, sedation, lightheadedness,** giddiness, vertigo, excitement, **numbness, tingling,** headache, amnesia
- □ May induce apnea if not self-administered

Other
- □ Expansion of gas filled pockets
- □ N/v, cyanosis

PRECAUTIONS:
1. Gas mixture may separate @ <-6°C[53]
2. Store & administer with cylinder horizontal
3. Confined spaces (may affect crew members)[54]
4. Severe maxillo-facial injuries (use mouthpiece)
5. Anytime >50% FiO_2 is required (d/c if cyanosis develops)

INTERACTIONS: None significant

[53]May also separate if cylinder pressure is too low (O_2 rises). If frost develops on tanks as they are used, change tanks. Do not use tank @ <6°C for >10 min. Rewarm @ room temperature for 24 hr.
[54]Especially if venting is inadequate.

NITROUS OXIDE/OXYGEN

CONTRA-INDICATIONS:

1. Impaired LOC from any source
2. Chest trauma (actual or potential pneumothorax)
3. Inability to comply with instructions
4. Cyanosis during use
5. Decompression sickness (bends), nitrogen narcosis, air emboli, air transport
6. Undiagnosed abdominal pain, marked distention, known bowel obstruction
7. Hypotension/shock

PREPARATIONS: D & E cylinders (blue & white in Canada, blue & green in U.S.) of 50% N_2O : 50% O_2 compressed gas

DOSE:

Adult Invert 3× before use (6× if <10°C)
Self-administered by normal, deep inhalation, via demand valve & mask (or mouthpiece)

Child Same as adult

SPECIAL:

1. Also known as "laughing gas," "N_2O : O_2"
2. May not provide total pain relief. May have no effect on some people

ORCIPRENOLINE (METAPROTERENOL) — Alupent (Metaprel)

TYPE: **Bronchodilator (Sympathomimetic)**

ACTIONS:

1. Selective β_2 stimulation → bronchodilation (& some peripheral vasodilation)
2. Some β_1 & little or no α-stimulation

	Onset	Peak	Duration
Aerosol	5-15 min	60-90 min	1-5 hr
Nebulized	5-15 min	60-90 min	1-6 hr

INDICATIONS & USES: Bronchospasm (associated with asthma, chronic bronchitis, or emphysema)

ADVERSE EFFECTS:

CVS
- □ Tachycardia, palpitation, hypertension, angina, PVCs, arrhythmia

CNS
- □ Nervousness, weakness, drowsiness, dizziness, tremor, headache

Other
- □ Bad taste, n/v
- □ May cause severe paradoxical bronchospasm from repeated excessive use

PRECAUTIONS: Cardiovascular disorders

INTERACTIONS: β-blockers: inhibit effects

CONTRA-INDICATIONS: Tachyarrhythmia

PREPARATIONS:

65 μg/metered dose aerosol inhaler
75 μg/metered dose aerosol inhaler
90 μg/metered dose aerosol inhaler
50 mg/10 ml bottle nebulizer solution (5 mg/ml) 0.5%

Alupent (Metaprel) — ORCIPRENOLINE (METAPROTERENOL)

DOSE:

Adult ***Aerosol*** 2-3 inhalations
Repeat q 15 min, p.r.n.
Nebulized 2.5-5 mg (0.5-1 ml) in 3-4 ml NS
Repeat p.r.n.

Child ***Aerosol*** 1-2 inhalations
Repeat q 15 min, p.r.n.
Nebulized 0.15 mg (0.03 ml)/kg in 3-4 ml NS
Repeat p.r.n.

Note: May also dilute nebulizer solution in sterile H_2O.

SPECIAL:

1. Also a common prescription drug
2. β_2 selectivity is lost with high doses

OXYGEN

TYPE: **Naturally occurring atmospheric gas (21% in air)**

ACTIONS:
1. Increases pO_2 → reverses hypoxemia
2. Oxidizes glucose to produce ATP
3. May reduce the size of (or eliminate) infarct during AMI

	Onset	Peak	Duration
Inhale	Immediate	<1 min	<2 min

INDICATIONS & USES:
1. Prevention/Tx of hypoxemia (global or local) from any cause (drug of choice)
2. All patients with acute ischemic chest pain
3. Any critical patient
4. Prophylactically in most patients during flight
5. Any respiratory difficulty

ADVERSE EFFECTS:
- None with short-term use (<24 hr) in adults

PRECAUTIONS:
1. COPD patients with CO_2 retention.[55] ***Never withhold*** **high FiO_2 & flow rates *if required***
2. Neonates → drastic pO_2 changes can cause blindness (retrolental fibroplasia)
3. Children → excessive (+) pressure ventilation may create a pneumothorax

INTERACTIONS: None significant

CONTRA-INDICATIONS: None significant

PREPARATIONS: D & E cylinders (usually green & white) of 100% O_2 compressed gas

DOSE:

Adult Depends on condition being treated. Any critical patient should receive 100% FiO_2.

Child Same as adult

[55]High FiO_2 & flow rates *infrequently* cause decreased LOC & respiratory depression (however, be prepared to ventilate).

Method	Flow rate (1pm)	FiO_2 (%)*
Nasal prongs	1-6†	24-44
Nebulizing mask	5-6	40
Venturi mask	4-12	24-50
Simple mask	6-10‡	40-60
Partial rebreathing	6-10‡	35-60
Nonrebreathing	6-10‡	60-95
Mouth-mask	10-15	50-80
Bag-valve-mask (with reservoir bag)	10-15	40-90
Bag-valve-ETT (with reservoir)	10-15	100
(without reservoir)	10-15	40-50

*Also dependent upon tidal volume & respiratory rate.
†Flows >6 L/min cause rapid drying & dehydration of nasal mucosa & do not significantly increase FiO_2.
‡Lower flow rates cause CO_2 retention.

SPECIAL:

1. Also known as "O_2"
2. Also a common home drug

Chart of Common O_2 Cylinders

Name	Volume (liters)	Factor
M	3000	1.42
E	660	0.28
D	400	0.16

$$\textbf{Cylinder time} = \frac{[\text{gauge pressure} - 200\ (\text{psi})] \times \text{Cylinder factor}}{\text{Flow rate (lpm)}}$$

OXYTOCIN

Syntocinon
Pitocin

TYPE: **Oxytocic**

ACTIONS:
1. Stimulates uterine smooth muscle to contract
2. Uterine vasoconstriction
3. Stimulates lactation

	Onset	Peak	Duration
IV IM	<1 min 3-7 min		2-3 min 2-3 hr

INDICATIONS & USES: Postpartum hemorrhage *after* infant & placental delivery

ADVERSE EFFECTS:

CVS
- □ Hypotension, tachycardia
- □ Hypertension, arrhythmia, PVCs, angina

CNS
- □ Anxiety, seizure

Other
- □ N/v, allergic reaction, dyspnea
- □ Uterine hypertonic spasms/contractions, rupture

PRECAUTIONS:
1. May cause placental retention if given prior to placental delivery
2. Hx of C-section or uterine surgery
3. Traumatic delivery

INTERACTIONS: Other vasopressors: potentiate hypertension

CONTRA-INDICATIONS: Presence of a 2nd fetus

PREPARATIONS:
10 USP units/1 ml ampule (10 U/ml)
5 USP units/1 ml ampule (5 U/ml)

DOSE: **Adult** 5-20 U/500 ml LR (or NS), IV infusion @ 20-40 mU/min *or* 5-10 U IM
Increase p.r.n., to control bleeding (uterine tone)

SPECIAL: Commonly used in conjunction with:
a. Fluid replacement
b. Uterine massage
c. PASG
d. Suckling

More common in interhospital use

TYPE: **Neuromuscular Blocker (nondepolarizing)**

ACTIONS: Blocks depolarization → skeletal muscle relaxation & paralysis

	Onset	Peak	Duration
IV	<1 min	3-5 min	30-90 min

INDICATIONS & USES: Induction or maintenance of paralysis post ETT (to assist with ventilation)

> **Note:** Paralyzation should ***always*** be preceded with an ETT in out-of-hospital care.

ADVERSE EFFECTS:

CVS
- Possible transient hypotension
- **Tachycardia,** arrhythmia, PVCs, ↑ BP

Other
- Excessive salivation
- Pain, burning at IV site

PRECAUTIONS:
1. Cardiovascular, hepatic, or renal insufficiency
2. Neuromuscular disease (e.g., myasthenia gravis)
3. Does *not* stop neuronal seizure activity (which may be undetectable in a paralyzed patient)

INTERACTIONS: (+) chronotropics: potentiate tachycardia

CONTRA-INDICATIONS:
1. When ↑ HR may be undesirable
2. Anyone in whom you do not have airway control & (+) pressure ventilation with O_2

PREPARATIONS: 4 mg/2 ml ampule (2 mg/ml)

PANCURONIUM — Pavulon

More common in interhospital use

DOSE:

> **Note:** Induce unconsciousness (if conscious) prior to paralyzing patient.[56]
> **Note:** Allow effects of "Succ" to diminish before giving Pancuronium.

	Adult	0.1 mg/kg slow IV Repeat q 30-60 min, p.r.n.
	Child	Same as adult
SPECIAL:		May be reversed by Neostigmine (Prostigmin) & should be accompanied by Atropine (0.6-1.2 mg IV)

[56]Has no effect on consciousness or pain.

More common in interhospital use

TYPE: **Anticonvulsant, Sedative-Hypnotic**

ACTIONS:
1. Suppresses (limits) spread of seizure activity & raises the seizure threshold (in the motor cortex)
2. Depresses the CNS

	Onset	Peak	Duration
IV IM	3-30 min	<30 min	4-6 hr 4-6 hr

INDICATIONS & USES:
1. Prevention/Tx of seizure activity (refractory to Diazepam)
2. Prophylactically (postseizure activity)
3. Anxiety, apprehension

ADVERSE EFFECTS:

CVS
- **Hypotension,**[57] bradycardia

CNS
- **Respiratory depression,**[58] **CNS depression, drowsiness, dizziness,** ataxia, **"hangover,"** coma
- Occasional paradoxical CNS stimulation (especially in children & the elderly)

Other
- Warmth, pain, burning, or phlebitis extending from IV site, thrombosis
- N/v, pupil constriction, nystagmus

PRECAUTIONS:
1. Extravasation may cause tissue necrosis
2. Pulmonary, cardiovascular, hepatic, or renal insufficiency

INTERACTIONS: Other anticonvulsants, CNS depressants, MAOIs: may potentiate effects

CONTRA-INDICATIONS: Hypoglycemic seizure (use Dextrose)

[57]Especially if given too rapidly. Be prepared to resuscitate.
[58]See footnote 57.

PHENOBARBITAL — Luminal

More common in interhospital use

PREPARATIONS:		120 mg/1 ml ampule (120 mg/ml) 130 mg/2 ml vial (65 mg/ml)
DOSE:	**Adult**	1-5 mg/kg (diluted) slow IV @ <60 mg/min (or IM) Repeat q 10-30 min, MAX 20 mg/kg
	Child	15-20 mg/kg (diluted) slow IV @ <30 mg/min (or IM, PR) Maintenance infusion 4 mg/kg q12h
SPECIAL:		Also a common prescription drug

More common in interhospital use

TYPE: **Anticonvulsant, Antiarrhythmic (class Ib)**

ACTIONS:

1. Suppresses (limits) spread of seizure activity & raises the seizure threshold (in the motor cortex)
2. (−) inotrope, depresses automaticity
3. (+) dromotrope (especially when "Dig" depressed), prolongs refractory period

	Onset	Peak	Duration
IV	3-5 min	1-2 hr	Long

Note: Slower onset & longer duration than Diazepam.

INDICATIONS & USES:

1. Prevention/Tx of seizure activity (refractory to Diazepam)
2. Prophylactically (postseizure activity) (drug of choice)
3. Refractory "Dig"-induced arrhythmias

ADVERSE EFFECTS:

CVS
- **Hypotension,[59] arrhythmia[60]**

CNS
- **Respiratory depression,[61] CNS depression, ataxia, slurred speech, confusion,** headache, drowsiness, dizziness, nervousness, tremor

Other
- Warmth, pain, burning, or phlebitis extending from IV site
- N/v, nystagmus, visual disturbances

PRECAUTIONS:

1. Extravasation may cause tissue necrosis
2. Cardiovascular, hepatic, or renal insufficiency
3. Rather insoluble & may precipitate in solutions other than NS

---

[59]Especially if given too rapidly. Be prepared to resuscitate.
[60]See footnote 59.
[61] See footnote 59.

PHENYTOIN — Dilantin

More common in interhospital use

INTERACTIONS:
1. Anticoagulants, other anticonvulsants, Diazoxide, salicylates: may potentiate effects
2. Sympathomimetics: sudden hypotension/bradycardia

CONTRA-INDICATIONS:
1. Hypoglycemic seizure (use Dextrose)
2. Bradycardia, 2° or 3° AV block

PREPARATIONS:
100 mg/2 ml ampule (50 mg/ml)
250 mg/5 ml ampule (50 mg/ml)

DOSE:

> **Note:** Dilute only in NS. Should use an in-line filter.

Adult ***Seizures:***
15-20 mg/kg, IV infusion minibag @ <50 mg/min (elderly @ <50 mg over 2-3 min), MAX 2 g
Arrhythmias:
50-100 mg (diluted) slow IV @ <50 mg/min
Repeat q 5-15 min, p.r.n., MAX 1 g

> **Note:** Mean adult lethal dose is about 2-5 g.

Child 10-20 mg/kg, IV infusion @ 1 mg/kg/min

> **Note:** Flush to avoid precipitation.

SPECIAL:
1. Also a common prescription drug
2. May normally have a slight yellow color

TYPE: **Antiarrhythmic (class Ia)**

ACTIONS:

1. Suppresses PVCs
2. Suppresses reentry arrhythmias
3. May elevate the threshold for VF
4. (−) chronotrope
5. (−) dromotrope
6. Mild (−) inotrope
7. Potent peripheral vasodilation

	Onset	Peak	Duration
IV	10-30 min	15-60 min	3-6 hr

INDICATIONS & USES:

1. PVCs (refractory to Lidocaine)
2. VT with pulse (refractory to Lidocaine)
3. PSVTs, wide complex tachycardia of unknown origin (drug of choice when associated with WPW)

ADVERSE EFFECTS:

CVS □ **Hypotension, bradycardia,** reflex tachycardia, AV block, widened QRS, prolonged PR or QT, PVCs, other conduction disturbances, arrhythmia (VT, VF, asystole)

CNS □ CNS depression, hallucination, confusion, dizziness, seizure

Other □ **N/v,** fever

PRECAUTIONS:

1. Asthma, AMI, "Dig"-induced arrhythmias
2. Cardiac, hepatic, or renal insufficiency
3. A-fib or A-flutter (may increase v-rate)

INTERACTIONS: None significant

CONTRA-INDICATIONS:

1. 3° AV blocks
2. "Dig"-toxicity
3. TCA-induced arrhythmia
4. Atypical VT (torsades de pointes)

PREPARATIONS: 1 g/10 ml vial (100 mg/ml)

DOSE:

Adult 50 mg slow IV @ <20 mg/min
Repeat q 5 min, p.r.n.,[62] MAX 1 g
IV infusion 1 g/250 ml @ 1-4 mg/min

Child Safety & efficacy not well established

Note: *Cardiac arrest:* Use bolus therapy only. After resuscitation, consider infusion.
Recurrent arrhythmia or PVCs: Repeat bolus & increase infusion rate by 1 mg/min.
Prevention: Bolus & follow with infusion.

SPECIAL: Also a common prescription drug

IV INFUSION DOSAGE/FLOW RATE CHART

For a **1 g/250 ml** solution **(4 mg/ml)**

Desired dose (mg/min)	Flow rate (ml/hr)
1	15
2	30
3	45
4	60

[62]Until the arrhythmia is suppressed, hypotension develops, the QRS widens by 50% of original, or other toxic signs appear (usually effective by 500-600 mg).

More common in interhospital use

TYPE: **β-Blocker, Antiarrhythmic (class II)**

ACTIONS: β_1 & β_2 receptor blockade (non-selective)

	Onset	Peak	Duration
IV	<2 min	15 min	2-6 hr

INDICATIONS & USES:
1. Reflex tachycardia[63]
2. Hypertension[64]
3. Post-MI (for recurrent tachyarrhythmia)

ADVERSE EFFECTS:
- **CVS** □ **Hypotension, bradycardia,** AV block, **may precipitate CHF,** angina
- **Other** □ **May precipitate *severe* bronchospasm (in COPD)**

PRECAUTIONS:
1. may be critically dependent on β-stimulation
2. Can mask signs of shock & hypoglycemia
3. "Dig"-induced arrhythmias, WPW

INTERACTIONS:
1. Cardiac depressants: potentiate bradycardia & myocardial depression
2. Sympathomimetics, Aminophylline, Glucagon, Atropine: may oppose some effects
3. "Epi": severe vasoconstriction

CONTRA-INDICATIONS:
1. Asthmatics, COPD, or any potential bronchospasm
2. Any depressed cardiac function

PREPARATIONS: 1 mg/1 ml ampule, vial (1 mg/ml)

DOSE:
- **Adult** 1-3 mg (diluted) slow IV @ <1 mg/min
  Repeat after 5-10 min, p.r.n., MAX 0.1 mg/kg
- **Child** 0.01-0.05 mg/kg (diluted) slow IV over 10 min
  Repeat q 5-10 min, p.r.n., MAX 3 mg

SPECIAL:
1. Also a common prescription drug
2. Cardioversion may cause asystole

---

[63]As an adjunct to potent vasodilators, to prevent or treat reflex tachycardia (from excessive sympathetic stimulation).
[64]See footnote 63.

RACEMIC EPINEPHRINE

Vaponefrin
Micronefrin

TYPE: **Bronchodilator (Sympathomimetic)**

ACTIONS:
1. Bronchodilation
2. (+) chromotropic
3. (+) inotropic

Onset	Peak	Duration

INDICATIONS & USES:
1. Bronchospasm (due to asthma, hay fever, croup, bronchitis, emphysema, or other pulmonary disease)

Note: Used primarily in children with upper airway problems

ADVERSE EFFECTS:

CVS
- □ Tachycardia, hypertension, palpitation, angina, arrhythmia

CNS
- □ Tremor, nervousness, anxiety, dizziness, headache

Other
- □ Bronchial edema/inflammation
- □ Nausea, sweating
- □ May cause severe paradoxical bronchospasm from repeated excessive use

PRECAUTIONS: Hypertension, cardiovascular disorders

INTERACTIONS:
1. β-blockers: may inhibit beta effects
2. TCAs, MAOIs: may induce hypertensive crisis

CONTRA-INDICATIONS:
1. Patients with potential for tachyarrhythmias
2. Epiglottitis

PREPARATIONS: 30 ml bottle (2.25% solution) for nebulization

DOSE:

Adult ***Nebulized*** 0.5 ml in 3-4 ml NS
Repeat after 5 min, p.r.n., x1 only

Child Same as adult

SPECIAL:
1. May turn sputum a pink color

Ventolin (Proventil) — SALBUTAMOL (ALBUTEROL)

TYPE: **Bronchodilator (Sympathomimetic)**

ACTIONS:
1. Selective β_2 stimulation → bronchodilation (& some peripheral vasodilation)
2. Some β_1 & little or no α-stimulation

	Onset	Peak	Duration
Aerosol	5-15 min	30 min-3 hr	3-6 hr
Nebulized	5-15 min	30 min-3 hr	3-6 hr

INDICATIONS & USES: Bronchospasm (associated with asthma, chronic bronchitis, or emphysema)

ADVERSE EFFECTS:

CVS
- □ Tachycardia, palpitation, hypertension, angina, PVCs, arrhythmia
- □ Possible hypotension

CNS
- □ **Nervousness,** anxiety, **tremor, dizziness,** weakness, headache, sweating

Other
- □ Bad taste, n/v, muscle cramps, dry nose & throat
- □ May cause severe paradoxical bronchospasm from repeated excessive use

PRECAUTIONS: Cardiovascular disorders

INTERACTIONS: β-blockers: inhibit effects

CONTRA-INDICATIONS: Tachyarrhythmia

PREPARATIONS:
100 μg/metered dose aerosol inhaler
90 μg/metered dose aerosol inhaler
50 mg/10 ml bottle, nebulizer sol'n (5 mg/ml) 0.5%
2.5 mg/2.5 ml ampule, nebulizer sol'n (1 mg/1 ml)

SALBUTAMOL (ALBUTEROL) — Ventolin (Proventil)

DOSE:

Adult ***Aerosol*** 2-3 inhalations
Repeat q 15 min, p.r.n.
Nebulized 1.5-5 mg (0.25-1 ml) in 3-4 ml NS
Repeat p.r.n.

Child ***Aerosol*** 1-2 inhalations
Repeat q 15 min, p.r.n.
Nebulized 0.15 mg (0.03 ml)/kg in 3-4 ml NS
Repeat p.r.n.

Note: May also dilute nebulizer solution in sterile H_2O.

SPECIAL:

1. Also a common prescription drug
2. β_2 selectivity is lost with high doses

TYPE: **Alkalinizing Agent ("buffer")**

ACTIONS: Buffers or neutralizes excess acid

	Onset	Peak	Duration
IV	<15 min		Depends on ongoing cause of metabolic acidosis

INDICATIONS & USES: *Metabolic* acidosis (cardiac arrest)[65]

ADVERSE EFFECTS: **Other**
- **Metabolic alkalosis**
- Hypoxia (indirect inhibition of O_2 release)
- Paradoxical rise in intracellular pCO_2
- Electrolyte imbalance, tetany
- May precipitate seizures or arrhythmias
- May cause ICH in infants

PRECAUTIONS: Extravasation causes tissue necrosis

INTERACTIONS:
1. Catecholamines: may inactivate
2. Ca^{++} salts: precipitates, turns to "chalk"

CONTRA-INDICATIONS:
1. Early in an arrest
2. Suspected metabolic alkalosis

PREPARATIONS:
50 mEq/50 ml preload (1 mEq/ml) 8.4%
44.6 mEq/50 ml preload (0.9 mEq/ml) 7.5%
5 mEq/10 ml preload (0.5 mEq/ml) 4.2%

DOSE:

Adult 1 mEq/kg slow IV
Repeat 0.5 mEq/kg q 10-15 min, p.r.n.

Child 1-3 mEq/kg slow IV (or IO), MAX 50 mEq
Repeat 0.5 mEq/kg q 10-15 min, p.r.n.

Infant 1-2 mEq/kg (4.2%) very slow IV (or IO) @ <1 mEq/kg/min *or* (1 mEq/kg of 8.4%, diluted 1:1), MAX 50 mEq
Repeat 0.5 mEq/kg q 10-15 min, p.r.n.

[65]Controversial; should only be used in a prolonged arrest (>5-10 min) after more proven treatments have been used.

SODIUM BICARBONATE

SPECIAL:

1. Also known as "Bicarb", "$NaHCO_3$"
2. "Bicarb" is an alkaline (base) solution

INTERHOSPITAL CONSIDERATIONS

Indications & Uses:

1. Metabolic acidosis:[66]
   a. Cardiac arrest[67]
   b. Other severe hypoperfusion states or acidosis[68]
2. Severe preexisting hypercalcemia
3. Hyperkalemia

Dose: In the absence of ABG results:

Adult (as above) or IV infusion 2-5 mEq/kg over 4-8 hr

Child (as above) or IV infusion 2-5 mEq/kg over 4-8 hr

Infant (as above)

---

[66]Usually only in severe acidosis (pH <7.1-7.2) or when the cause cannot be corrected by other more proven means. Complete correction with $NaHCO_3$ alone is dangerous & may be unnecessary.
[67]Ideally governed by ABG analysis (which is also controversial). Generally, correct pH toward normal (7.25-7.35 is generally acceptable), initially with 33-50% of the calculated HCO_3^-, & allow compensatory mechanisms to complete the correction. See also footnote 66.
[68]E.g., salicylate, barbiturate, or tricyclic OD.

Streptase
Kabikinase

STREPTOKINASE

More common in interhospital use

TYPE: **Fibrinolytic/Thrombolytic**

ACTIONS: "Dissolves" the thrombus (clot)

> **Note:** Dissolves all clots (nonselective). Systemic lysis.

	Onset	Peak	Duration
IV	Usually <1 hr	≃80 min	2-36 hr

INDICATIONS & USES: Evolving AMI, ideally within 1½ hr (but up to 4-6 hr) from onset

> **Note:** Refer to local protocol for patient suitability.

ADVERSE EFFECTS:

CVS
- ☐ Spontaneous **minor bleeding**[69] to severe hemorrhage
- ☐ Hypotension, reperfusion arrhythmias[70]

Other
- ☐ **Phlebitis** at injection site
- ☐ Allergic reaction,[71] mild **fever,**[72] nausea

PRECAUTIONS: Seriously consider benefits versus risks:

1. Internal hemorrhage may be difficult to control; examine regularly for signs of bleeding
2. Fibrin deposits that provide hemostasis (e.g., needle puncture sites)
3. Avoid unnecessary vessel puncture, central lines; use small-gauge needle
4. Minimize patient handling
5. Severe hepatic or renal insufficiency, >75 yr

INTERACTIONS:

1. Anticoagulants, anti-PLTs: may increase risk of bleeding
2. Dextrans: incompatible

---

[69]Oozing from vessel puncture is common.
[70]Commonly: accelerated A-fib, IVR, VT, SB, 2° or 3° AV block, or PVCs, which usually respond well to therapy. **Note:** Some suggest prophylactic Lidocaine.
[71]May be premedicated with Solu-Cortef, Benadryl, or Tylenol to minimize allergic or pyrogenic reaction.
[72]See footnote 71.

STREPTOKINASE

Streptase
Kabikinase

More common in interhospital use

CONTRA-INDICATIONS:
1. Almost any predisposition to bleeding
2. Severe hypertension
3. IM injection

PREPARATIONS: 250,000 IU (green label) white powder/6.5 ml vial
750,000 IU (blue label) white powder/6.5 ml vial
Reconstitute: With 5 ml NS (or D_5W). Do not vent vial of undissolved powder. Inject slowly along side of vial. Roll & tilt gently; *do not shake.* May foam or flocculate slightly; let stand. Discard if heavy.

DOSE:[73]

> **Note:** Should be infused through a 0.22 micron filter

Adult 1.5 million IU in 100 ml, IV infusion
Loading (750,000 IU) 5 ml/min for 10 min, then,
Maintenance (750,000 IU) 1 ml/min for 50 min

> **Note:** Some suggest following "SK" with a Heparin infusion to prevent re-thrombosis.

Child Safety & efficacy not yet established

SPECIAL:
1. Also known as "SK"
2. May be reversed by Aminocaproic Acid (Amicar)

[73]Obtain coagulation times (PT, PTT) prior to administration.

More common in interhospital use

TYPE: **Neuromuscular Blocker (depolarizing)**

ACTIONS: Inhibits/prolongs neuromuscular transmission → skeletal muscle relaxation & paralysis

	Onset	Peak	Duration
IV	<1 min	2 min	4-10 min

INDICATIONS & USES: To facilitate intubation (drug of choice)

ADVERSE EFFECTS:

CVS
- □ Hypotension, **bradycardia, arrhythmia**
- □ Hypertension, tachycardia

CNS
- □ **Initial muscle fasciculation,** excessive salivation,[74] bronchospasm

Other
- □ **Malignant hyperthermia**[75]
- □ Allergic reaction, may induce hyperkalemia

PRECAUTIONS:

1. Renal insufficiency
2. When histamine release may be hazardous
3. Severe asthma, neuromuscular disease (e.g., myasthenia gravis)
4. Severe burns, trauma (unstable fracture, spinal injury)
5. Does *not* stop neuronal seizure activity (which may be undetectable in a paralyzed patient)
6. Fasciculations may cause vomiting

---

[74]May be controlled by pretreatment with Atropine.

[75]Early signs: failure to relax (i.e., lack of laryngeal relaxation & general rigidity), tachycardia, hypertension, hyperventilation.

More common in interhospital use

INTERACTIONS:

1. Oxytocin, β-blockers, organophosphates: may potentiate some effects
2. Diazepam: may reduce duration of action
3. Cardiac glycosides: may induce arrhythmias

CONTRA-INDICATIONS: Penetrating eye injury[76]

PREPARATIONS: 40 mg/2 ml ampule (20 mg/ml)
100 mg/5 ml ampule (20 mg/ml)

DOSE:

> **Note:** Induce unconsciousness (if conscious) prior to paralyzing patient.[77] Consider premedication with Atropine.

Adult 1.5 mg/kg rapid IV
Repeat p.r.n., ×1 (use Atropine with repeat doses)

Child 1-2 mg/kg rapid IV
Repeat p.r.n., ×1

> **Note:** Young children may be less sensitive than adults & may require a slightly higher initial dose.

SPECIAL:

1. Also known as "Succ"
2. Should not be used without great confidence of performing a successful intubation

---

[76]Causes a slight increase in intraocular pressure (Pancuronium & Vecuronium do not).
[77]Has no effect on consciousness or pain.

TYPE: **Vitamin B_1**

ACTIONS: Essential for normal breakdown of glucose

	Onset	Peak	Duration
IV	Rapid		Depends on degree of deficiency

Note: Neurological improvements within a few hours.

INDICATIONS & USES: As conjunctive therapy with $D_{50}W$[78] in coma of unknown origin (especially if alcoholism or malnourishment is suspected)

ADVERSE EFFECTS:

CVS
- **Hypotension** (from rapid IV injection or large doses)

CNS
- Feeling of warmth, sweating
- Anxiety, weakness

Other
- Possible severe allergic reaction (especially if given too fast)
- Nausea

PRECAUTIONS: Severe allergic reaction can occur

INTERACTIONS: None significant

CONTRA-INDICATIONS: None significant

PREPARATIONS: 1000 mg/10 ml vial (100 mg/ml)

DOSE:

Adult 100 mg (diluted) very slow IV over 2-5 min (or IV infusion, IM)

Child Uncommon

SPECIAL: Also sometimes used for a "rare" type of myocardial failure called beriberi

[78]To prevent or treat thiamine deficiency (which may lead to Wernicke's encephalopathy).

rt-PA
ALTEPLASE — Activase

More common in interhospital use

TYPE: **Fibrinolytic/Thrombolytic (a recombinant tissue plasminogen activator "rt-PA")**

ACTIONS: "Dissolves" the thrombus (clot)

> **Note:** Dissolves recently formed clots (selective). Lysis at the site of the clot.

	Onset	Peak	Duration
IV	<90 min		5-10 min

INDICATIONS & USES: Evolving AMI, ideally within 1½ hr (but up to 4-6 hr) from onset

> **Note:** Refer to local protocol for patient suitability.

ADVERSE EFFECTS:

CVS
- □ Spontaneous **minor bleeding**[79] to severe hemorrhage
- □ Hypotension, reperfusion arrhythmias[80]

Other
- □ N/v, fever

PRECAUTIONS: Seriously consider benefits versus risks:
1. Internal hemorrhage may be difficult to control; examine regularly for signs of bleeding
2. Fibrin deposits that provide hemostasis (e.g., needle puncture sites)
3. Avoid unnecessary vessel puncture, central lines; use small-gauge needle
4. Minimize patient handling
5. Severe hepatic or renal insufficiency, >75 yr

INTERACTIONS:
1. Anticoagulants, anti-PLTs: may increase risk of bleeding
2. Dextrans: incompatible

CONTRA-INDICATIONS:
1. Almost any predisposition to bleeding
2. Severe hypertension
3. IM injection

---

[79] Oozing from vessel puncture is common.

[80] Commonly: accelerated A-fib, IVR, VT, SB, 2° or 3° AV block, or PVCs, which usually respond well to therapy. **Note:** Some suggest prophylactic Lidocaine.

More common in interhospital use

PREPARATIONS:

20 mg (white powder)/20 ml vial
50 mg (white powder)/50 ml vial
Supplied with Sterile Water for Injection USP without preservatives (20 & 50 ml vials)
Reconstitute: *Only* with diluent provided (1 mg/ml). Do not vent vial of undissolved powder. Inject slowly along side of vial. Roll & tilt gently; *do not shake.* May foam or flocculate slightly; let stand. Add to *empty* 100 ml mini-bag.

DOSE:[81]

> **Note:** Should be infused through a 0.22 micron filter.

Adult 1.25-1.5 mg/kg (≅ 100 mg, MAX 120 mg)
Loading 6-10 mg slow IV over 4-10 min, then,
Maintenance 0.75 mg/kg IV infusion over 1 hr, then,
0.25 mg/kg IV infusion over 1 hr

> **Note:** Some suggest using a Heparin infusion concomitantly & following "TPA" termination to prevent rethrombosis.

Child Safety & efficacy not yet established

SPECIAL:

1. May be reversed by Aminocaproic Acid (Amicar)
2. Also known as "TPA"

[81]Obtain coagulation times (PT, PTT) prior to administration.

More common in interhospital use

TYPE: **Neuromuscular Blocker (nondepolarizing)**

ACTIONS: Blocks depolarization → skeletal muscle relaxation & paralysis

	Onset	Peak	Duration
IV	2-3 min	3-5 min	25-40 min

INDICATIONS & USES: Induction or maintenance of paralysis post-ETT (to assist with ventilation)

> **Note:** Paralyzation should ***always*** be preceded with an ETT in out-of-hospital care.

ADVERSE EFFECTS: □ None significant

PRECAUTIONS:
1. Hepatic insufficiency
2. Neuromuscular disease (e.g., myasthenia gravis)
3. Does *not* stop neuronal seizure activity (which may be undetectable in a paralyzed patient)

INTERACTIONS: None significant

CONTRA-INDICATIONS: Anyone in whom you do not have airway control & (+) pressure ventilation with O_2

PREPARATIONS: 10 mg (powder)/5 ml vial
Reconstitute: With 5 ml Sterile Water for Injection (2 mg/ml)

DOSE:

> **Note:** Induce unconsciousness (if conscious) prior to paralyzing patient.[82]
> **Note:** Allow effects of "Succ" to diminish before giving Vecuronium.

[82]Has no effect on consciousness or pain.

More common in interhospital use

Adult 0.1 mg/kg rapid IV
Repeat q 25-40 min, p.r.n.

Child Same as adult

Note: Young children may be less sensitive than adults & may require a slightly higher initial dose.

SPECIAL:

1. May be reversed by Neostigmine (Prostigmin) & should be accompanied by Atropine (0.6-1.2 mg IV)
2. Unlike other nondepolarizing neuromuscular blockers, Vecuronium has no effect on the CVS & does not cause histamine release

VERAPAMIL

Isoptin Calan

TYPE: **Calcium (slow) Channel Blocker**
Antiarrhythmic (class IV)

ACTIONS: Blocks entry of Ca^{++} into cells (especially cardiac & vascular smooth muscle) →:

a. (−) dromotropy & depresses atrial automaticity[83]
b. (−) chronotropy
c. (−) inotropy
d. Vasodilation (including coronary)

IV	Onset	Peak	Duration
AV node	<5 min	<15 min	30-60 min
Hemodynamic	4-6 min	<5 min	10-20 min

INDICATIONS & USES: Symptomatic (narrow complex) SVTs that:

a. Do not require immediate cardioversion
b. Are refractory to vagal maneuvers

ADVERSE EFFECTS:[84]

CVS
- **Hypotension,** bradycardia, AV or sinus blocks, asystole, VF; flushing
- May induce or exacerbate CHF/pulmonary edema

CNS
- Headache, dizziness, sweating, seizure

Other
- N/v, abdominal pain

PRECAUTIONS:

1. Cardiovascular, hepatic, or renal insufficiency
2. Use with anything that slows AV conduction or depresses myocardial function
3. Wide complex tachycardia
4. Proximate cardioversion may induce bradycardia

INTERACTIONS: β-blockers: may potentiate effects → heart failure

[83] Interrupts reentry pathways & slows ventricular response.
[84] $CaCl_2$ may in part prevent or reverse Verapamil-induced hypotension or other adverse effects.

CONTRA-INDICATIONS:

1. Cardiogenic shock, AMI
2. A-fib or A-flutter associated with a bypass tract; evidence of preexcitation
3. Conduction disturbances (unassisted by a ventricular pacemaker)

PREPARATIONS:

5 mg/2 ml ampule (2.5 mg/ml)
2 mg/2 ml ampule (1 mg/ml)

DOSE:

Adult 2-5 mg (0.1 mg/kg) slow IV (elderly @ 2 mg over 3-4 min), MAX 10 mg
Repeat after 30 min, p.r.n.

Child 0.1-0.3 mg/kg slow IV, MAX 10 mg/dose
Repeat after 30 min, p.r.n.

SPECIAL:

Also a common prescription drug

Section Three

IV Solutions
Blood Products

5% DEXTROSE (D_5W)

TYPE: **Hypotonic Sugar Solution of 5% Dextrose in Water**

ACTIONS: Source of glucose & H_2O

INDICATIONS & USES:

1. Diluent & vehicle for reconstitution, injection, or infusion of most drugs
2. Patients with actual or potential for volume overload (fluid of choice)
3. Patients requiring Na^+ restriction
4. Hypoglycemia

ADVERSE EFFECTS:

- □ H_2O intoxication, hyponatremia
- □ Hyperglycemia

PRECAUTIONS:

1. Children → danger of H_2O intoxication (D_5W dilutes Na^+ → child may seizure)
2. Head injury, diabetes

CONTRA-INDICATIONS: As a mainline for blood transfusion[85]

PREPARATIONS: 50 ml, 100 ml, 250 ml, 500 ml, 1 L bag

DOSE:

Adult IV infusion, titrate to desired effect
Usually TKO, via microdrip

Child Same as adult

SPECIAL: Contains:

a. 5 g Dextrose/100 ml
b. ≃ pH 4.0
c. ≃ 252 mOsm/ml
d. Glucose 250 mmol/L
e. Available energy 710 kJ/L

[85] Dextrose solutions are incompatible with blood products (glucose causes red cells to clump).

5% DEXTROSE and 0.2% SODIUM CHLORIDE (D_5.2 NS)

TYPE: **Hypotonic Sugar & Crystalloid Solution of 5% Dextrose & 0.2% Sodium Chloride in Water**

ACTIONS: Source of glucose, Na^+, Cl^-, & H_2O

INDICATIONS & USES:
1. Na^+ maintenance in pediatric patients[86] (solution of choice)
2. Pediatric[87] emergencies

ADVERSE EFFECTS:
- H_2O intoxication, hyponatremia
- Hyperglycemia

PRECAUTIONS: Diabetes

CONTRA-INDICATIONS: As a mainline for blood transfusion[88]

PREPARATIONS: 250 ml, 500 ml bag

DOSE: **Adult** IV infusion, titrate to desired effect

Child Same as adult

SPECIAL: Contains:
a. 5 g Dextrose/100 ml
b. 200 g NaCl/100 ml
c. $\simeq$ pH 4.0
d. $\simeq$ 321 mOsm/L
e. Na^+ 34 mmol/L
f. Cl^- 34 mmol/L
g. Glucose 250 mmol/L
h. Available energy 710 kJ/L

Note: Children require about the same Na^+/kg as an adult but more H_2O than an adult. The solution concentration required therefore contains less Na^+ (i.e., NS contains too much Na^+ for children).

---

[86]Approximately <2 yr of age.
[87]See footnote 86.
[88]Dextrose solutions are incompatible with blood products (glucose causes red cells to clump).

3.3% DEXTROSE and 0.3% SODIUM CHLORIDE (⅔–⅓)

TYPE: **Isotonic Sugar & Crystalloid Solution of 3.3% Dextrose & 0.3% Sodium Chloride in Water**

ACTIONS: Source of glucose, Na^+, Cl^-, & H_2O

INDICATIONS & USES:
1. Long-term nonspecific IV route maintenance (i.e., to keep a line available)
2. Na^+ replacement (in children)
3. Dehydration

ADVERSE EFFECTS:
- H_2O intoxication, hyponatremia
- Hyperglycemia

PRECAUTIONS: Diabetes

CONTRA-INDICATIONS: As a mainline for blood transfusion[89]

PREPARATIONS: 500 ml, 1000 ml bag

DOSE:
Adult IV infusion, titrate to desired effect
Child Same as adult

SPECIAL: Contains:
a. 3.3 g Dextrose/100 ml
b. 300 mg NaCl/100 ml
c. $\simeq$ pH 4.0
d. $\simeq$ 269 mOsm/ml
e. Na^+ 51 mmol/L
f. Cl^- 51 mmol/L
g. Glucose 170 mmol/L
h. Available energy 470 kJ/L

---

[89]Dextrose solutions are incompatible with blood products (glucose causes red cells to clump).

TYPE:		**Hypertonic Sugar Solution of 10% Dextrose in Water**
ACTIONS:		Source of glucose & H_2O
INDICATIONS & USES:		1. Hypoglycemia (especially children) 2. ETOH intoxication
ADVERSE EFFECTS:		□ H_2O intoxication, hyponatremia □ Hyperglycemia
PRECAUTIONS:		Diabetes
CONTRA-INDICATIONS:		As a mainline for blood transfusion[90]
PREPARATIONS:		250 ml, 500 ml bag
DOSE:	**Adult**	IV infusion, titrate to desired effect
	Child	IV infusion @ <2 ml/kg/hr Titrate to desired effect
SPECIAL:		Contains: a. 10 g Dextrose/100 ml b. ≃pH 4.0 c. ≃505 mOsm/L d. Glucose 500 mmol/L e. Available energy 1420 kJ/L

[90]Dextrose solutions are incompatible with blood products (glucose causes red cells to clump).

LACTATED RINGER'S ("LR")

TYPE: **Isotonic Crystalloid Solution**

ACTIONS:
1. Source of electrolytes & H_2O
2. Increases circulating volume

INDICATIONS & USES:
1. To restore intravascular volume
2. Initial fluid & electrolyte replacement in:
   a. Hypovolemia
   b. Dehydration
   c. Burns (fluid of choice)
3. Irrigation, cooling burns
4. Crush injuries (fluid of choice)

ADVERSE EFFECTS: □ Volume overload, CHF, pulmonary edema

PRECAUTIONS:
1. CHF, pulmonary edema
2. Impaired lactate metabolism states (e.g., liver disease, anoxia)
3. May induce hypothermia with multiple infusions

CONTRA-INDICATIONS: As a mainline for blood transfusion[91]

PREPARATIONS: 250 ml, 500 ml, 1 L bag

DOSE: **Adult** IV infusion, titrate to desired effect

Child Same as adult

> **Note:** Use large bore cannula & tubing for volume infusion.

> **Note:** For rapid volume replacement, use warmed "LR" if possible. (Warm only by proven methods.)

[91]Lactated Ringer's is incompatible with blood products ("LR" contains Ca^{++}, which promotes clotting).

SPECIAL:

1. Also known as Ringer's Lactate "RL"
2. Contains:
   a. 600 mg NaCl/100 ml
   b. 310 mg Na Lactate/100 ml
   c. 30 mg KCl/100 ml
   d. 20 mg $CaCl_2$/100 ml
   e. ≃pH 6.5
   f. ≃272 mOsm/L
   g. Na^+ 130 mmol/L
   h. Cl^- 109 mmol/L
   i. K^+ 4 mmol/L
   j. Ca^{++} 1.5 mmol/L
   k. Lactate 28 mmol/L

0.9% SODIUM CHLORIDE (0.9% NaCl) NORMAL SALINE ("NS")

TYPE: **Isotonic Crystalloid Solution**

ACTIONS:
1. Source of Na^+, Cl^-, & H_2O
2. Increases circulating volume

INDICATIONS & USES:
1. To restore intravascular volume
2. Initial fluid & electrolyte replacement in:
   a. Hypovolemia
   b. Dehydration, Na^+, & Cl^- depletion
   c. Burns
3. Head injury (solution of choice)
4. Irrigation, cooling burns
5. Diluent & vehicle for reconstitution, injection, or infusion of most drugs
6. To dilute or warm blood & as a mainline for blood transfusion (solution of choice)
7. Ketoacidosis, diabetes, septic shock, fresh H_2O drowning, crush injuries

ADVERSE EFFECTS:
- □ Volume overload, CHF, or pulmonary edema
- □ Diuresis, electrolyte depletion, & acid-base imbalance (following large infusions)

PRECAUTIONS:
1. Renal impairment, CHF, pulmonary edema
2. May induce hypothermia with multiple infusions
3. <2 yr of age[92]

CONTRA-INDICATIONS: Use of bacteriostatic NaCl injection containing benzyl alcohol (preservative) in neonates

PREPARATIONS: 50 ml, 100 ml, 250 ml, 500 ml, 1 L bag
10 ml vial (with or without preservative) for Injection USP 0.9%

---

[92]May cause electrolyte imbalance.

0.9% SODIUM CHLORIDE (0.9% NaCl) NORMAL SALINE ("NS")

DOSE: **Adult** IV infusion, titrate to desired effect

Child Same as adult

Note: Use large bore cannula & tubing for volume infusion.

Note: For rapid volume replacement, use warmed "NS" if possible. (Warm only by proven methods.)

SPECIAL: Contains:

a. 900 mg NaCl/100 ml
b. ≈pH 5.0
c. ≈308 mOsm/L
d. Na^+ 154 mmol/L
e. Cl^- 154 mmol/L

CHOOSING BLOOD PRODUCTS and ABO GROUP COMPATIBILITY

Component therapy is generally considered superior to the use of whole blood for most emergencies.

In extreme emergencies, if the patient ABO group is unknown, O^+ is generally given, unless the patient is female and less than about 45 years of age (potential childbearing), in which case O^- is generally given.

Choices Available

	Blood	Plasma	Availability
Unmatched	O^+, O^-	AB	Immediate
Group & type-specific	(see chart)		5-10 min
Cross-matched	(see chart)		About 1 hr

ABO Group Compatibility Chart

Patient (recipient)	Donor RED CELLS (in priority order)	Donor PLASMAS (in priority order)
O	O	O, A, B, AB
A	A, O	A, AB
B	B, O	B, AB
AB	AB, A, B, O	AB

When to Change

If >5-8 units of group O have been given, then stay with group O.

Otherwise, change to group & type-specific blood products when available.

BLOOD PRODUCTS—GENERAL INFORMATION

The following is a *general overview of most blood products* that have been derived from whole blood.

TYPE: **Colloid Solutions (Volume Expanders)**

ACTIONS: Increases circulating vascular volume

INDICATIONS & USES: Volume replacement, resulting from hypovolemia due to hemorrhagic shock

ADVERSE EFFECTS:

- □ Volume overload, CHF, pulmonary edema
- □ Transfusion reaction[93]
- □ Infectious agent or immunizing agent transmission
- □ Hyperkalemia following massive transfusion
- □ Microaggregates may cause pulmonary insufficiency following massive transfusion
- □ Pain @ IV site

PRECAUTIONS:

1. Should be ABO group & Rh type compatible (whenever possible)
2. IV mainline solution should be NS[94]
3. Should be given through a blood filter no larger than standard 170 μm pore size (& changed after 2-10 units, depending on filter type)
4. Administration set should also have an antimicrobial filter
5. CHF, pulmonary edema
6. Risk of air embolism, especially if administered under pressure
7. Infusion pumps or excessive pressure may cause hemolysis
8. Cold solution may induce arrhythmia, paradoxical hypotension, or hypothermia
9. Rewarming beyond 38°C can cause hemolysis (warm only with approved equipment & methods)
10. No medication should be added directly
11. Infiltration causes tissue necrosis

---

[93]Most (but not all) blood products can cause transfusion reaction; febrile, allergic, or hemolytic being the more common (their severe adverse effects are typically evident within minutes). The most common cause of transfusion reaction is clerical identity error.

[94]"LR" & Dextrose solutions are incompatible with blood products ("LR" contains Ca^{++}, which promotes clotting & glucose causes red cells to clump).

BLOOD PRODUCTS—GENERAL INFORMATION—cont'd

CONTRA-INDICATIONS:

1. Volume-overloaded patient or patients in whom a rapid increase in circulating volume may be harmful
2. With IV solutions other than NS[95]

PREPARATIONS: Unit (volume is variable[96]) bag, bottle

DOSE: IV infusion via NS route
Rate depends on clinical status & patient response
(Generally slowly at first, but if necessary may infuse as rapidly as tolerated)

Adult ***Hypovolemia:*** 250-500 ml
Repeat in 15-30 min, p.r.n.

Child ***Hypovolemia:*** 10-20 ml/kg
Repeat in 15-30 min, p.r.n.

Note: A unit should not hang for >2-4 hr.

SPECIAL:

1. Labeled for ABO group & for Rh type
2. Should be kept cold in transport (unless being infused)

---

[95]See footnote 94.

[96]Blood products (except Albumin) are processed by their mass. Their volumes are variable & are referred to by the unit.

TYPE: **Colloid Solution of Plasma-Volume Expander**

ACTIONS:
1. Contains all plasma proteins & coagulation factors[97]
2. Increases circulating vascular volume

INDICATIONS & USES:
1. During or after multiple (massive) or very rapid transfusion[98]
2. Replacement of all coagulation factors (especially labile factors)
3. Temporary volume expansion

> **Note:** "FP" can replace "FFP" for most clinical situations. "FP" or "FFP" should be used only when labile coagulation factors are specifically required.

ADVERSE EFFECTS:
- □ Same as for all blood products

PRECAUTIONS:
1. Same as for all blood products
2. Administer promptly after thawing (factors V & VIII deteriorate rapidly)

CONTRA-INDICATIONS: Same as for all blood products

PREPARATIONS: 1 unit (about 200 ml) bag

DOSE: See General Information

SPECIAL:
1. Also known as "FP" & "FFP"
2. Thawing requires about 20-30 min
3. Compatible with red cells & Albumin

---

[97]"FP" differs primarily from "FFP" in that it is not frozen as quickly after processing. "FP" therefore contains only about 50-75% of the original factors V & VIII.
[98]Replacement of coagulation factors.

PLATELET CONCENTRATE

TYPE: **Colloid Solution of Platelets (PLTs)**
(Contains a few WBCs, some plasma, & some RBCs)

ACTIONS: Assists in hemostasis

INDICATIONS & USES:
1. During massive blood transfusion[99]
2. Prevention/Tx of bleeding due to proven PLT function disorders[100]

ADVERSE EFFECTS: □ Same as for all blood products

PRECAUTIONS: Same as for all blood products

CONTRA-INDICATIONS:
1. Disseminated intravascular coagulation (DIC)[101] (controversial)
2. Same as for all blood products

PREPARATIONS: 1 pool (about 6-8 units of 30-50 ml/unit) bag

DOSE:

Adult See General Information
Generally 6-10 PLT packs for every 10 units of red cells transfused

Child 1 U/5 kg

Note: 1 unit PLT concentrate will raise PLT count by about 5-10 $\times 10^9$/L, 1 hr after infusion.

SPECIAL:
1. May administer unmatched PLTs when clinically necessary
2. Stored @ room temperature

---

[99]To prevent or treat a coagulopathy.
[100]Thrombocytopenia or thrombocytopathia (inadequate or abnormal PLT production).
[101]Infused PLTs may be destroyed just as rapidly as those of the patient.

TYPE: **Colloid Solution of Red Blood Cells-Volume Expander** (Contains some plasma, WBCs, & PLTs)

ACTIONS:
1. Increases O_2 carrying capacity (by increasing Hgb concentration)
2. Increases circulating vascular volume

INDICATIONS & USES: To provide a mechanism for the transport of O_2 & replacement of lost RBCs (product of choice):
1. Hemorrhagic hypovolemia
2. Various types of symptomatic anemia

ADVERSE EFFECTS: □ Same as for all blood products

PRECAUTIONS:
1. Massive transfusion[102]
2. Same as for all blood products

CONTRA-INDICATIONS: Same as for all blood products

PREPARATIONS: 1 unit (about 300 ml) bag
Reconstitute: With ≈50-100 ml "NS" to reduce viscosity & warm

DOSE: See General Information

SPECIAL:
1. Also known as "RCC", packed red cells, RBCs
2. Newborns should receive <5 day old red cells if possible (fresh units have lower K^+ levels)
3. Compatible with Plasma & Albumin

---

[102]Usually >100 ml blood/min requires supplemental Ca^{++}. Anticoagulants in banked blood bind with recipient's Ca^{++}. For every 500 ml of blood received, give about 0.2 g (2 ml of 10%) $CaCl_2$ into a nonblood line, MAX 2 g (20 ml).

Section Four

Tables and Charts

ADULT GLASGOW COMA SCALE (GCS)

Physical sign		Response	Points	Score
Eye opening		Spontaneous	4	
		To verbal stimuli	3	
		To painful stimuli	2	
		None	1	____
Best motor response (upper limb)		Obeys command	6	
	To pain	Localizes	5	
		Withdraws	4	
		Abnormal-flexion*	3	
		Abnormal-extension†	2	
		None	1	____
Best verbal response		Oriented	5	
		Confused	4	
		Inappropriate words	3	
		Nonspecific sounds	2	
		None	1	____
TOTAL		Apply this score to GCS portion of Trauma Score	3-15	____

Score: Possible 3-15, decreasing with injury severity

*Formerly known as decorticate rigidity.
†Formerly known as decerebrate rigidity.

Pupil scale in millimeters

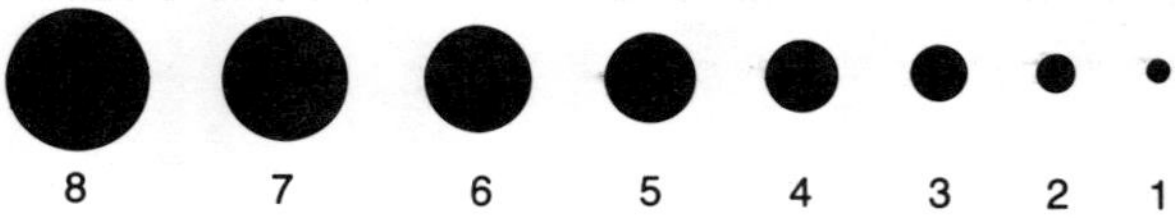

PEDIATRIC GLASGOW COMA SCALE (GCS)

Physical sign		Response	Response	Points	Score
		<1 Year	**>1 Year**		
Eye opening		Spontaneous	Spontaneous	4	
		To shout	To verbal stimuli	3	
		To pain	To pain	2	
		None	None	1	______
		<1 Year	**>1 Year**		
Best motor response (upper limb)		Normal spontaneous movements	Obeys commands	6	
	To pain	Localizes	Localizes	5	
		Withdraws	Withdraws	4	
		Abnormal-flexion*	Abnormal-flexion*	3	
		Abnormal-extension†	Abnormal-extension†	2	
		None	None	1	______
		<2 Years	**2-5 Years**		
Best verbal response		Smiles, coos, cries appropriately	Appropriate words & phrases	5	
		Appropriate cry	Inappropriate words	4	
		Inappropriate cry or scream	Cries or screams	3	
		Grunts/moans	Grunts	2	
		None	None	1	______
TOTAL				3-15	

Score: Possible 3-15, decreasing with injury severity

*Formerly known as decorticate rigidity.
†Formerly known as decerebrate rigidity.

ADULT PREHOSPITAL INDEX (PHI)

Physical sign	Value	Points	Score
Systolic BP (mmHg)	>100 86-100 75-85 <75	0 1 2 5	_____
Pulse rate (/min)	>120 51-120 <50	3 0 5	_____
Respiratory status	Normal Labored/shallow <10/min, needs ETT	0 3 5	_____
Level of consciousness	Normal Confused/combative No intelligible words	0 3 5	_____
TOTAL*		0-24	_____

Score: Possible 0-24, increasing with injury severity
Generally: 0-3 → minor trauma
4-24 → major trauma

*For penetrating abdominal or chest injuries, add 4 points to the total.

Physical sign	Value	Points	Score
Circulation	Capillary refill <2 sec & systolic BP >100	2	
	Capillary refill >2 sec *or* systolic BP 85-100	1	
	No capillary refill *or* systolic BP <85	0	____
Respirations	Normal	2	
	Labored or shallow	1	
	Absent	0	____
Abdomen, Thorax	Abdomen & thorax nontender	2	
	Abdomen *or* thorax tender	1	
	Abdomen rigid, flail chest, penetrating wound	0	____
Motor	Normal	2	
	Responds only to pain (other than decerebrate)	1	
	No response to pain *or* decerebrate	0	____
Speech	Normal	2	
	Confused	1	
	No intelligible words	0	____
TOTAL		0-10	____

Score: Possible 0-10, decreasing with injury severity
Generally: 9-10 → minor trauma
<9 → major trauma

ADULT TRAUMA SCORE (ATS)

Physical sign	Value	Points	Score
Respiratory rate (/min)	10-24 25-35 >35 <10 Apneic	4 3 2 1 0	______
Respiratory expansion (effort)	Normal Shallow Retractive	1 0 0	______
Systolic blood pressure (mmHg)	>90 70-90 50-69 <50 No Pulse	4 3 2 1 0	______
Capillary refill	Normal (<2 sec) Delayed (>2 sec) None	2 1 0	______
Glasgow Coma Scale (GCS)	14-15 11-13 8-10 5-7 3-4	5 4 3 2 1	______
TOTAL		1-16	______

Score: Possible 1-16, decreasing with injury severity
Generally: $>12 \rightarrow$ minor trauma
$<12 \rightarrow$ major trauma

PEDIATRIC TRAUMA SCORE (PTS)

Components	Points +2	Points +1	Points −1	Score
Weight	>20 kg (44 lb)	10-20 kg (22-44 lb)	<10 kg (<22 lb)	___
Airway	Patent*	Maintainable†	Unmaintainable‡	___
Systolic (cuff)	>90 mmHg	50-90 mmHg	<50 mmHg	
BP (pulses)	Radial	Femoral/carotid	None palpable	___
CNS	Awake, no ↓ LOC	Obtunded, some ↓ LOC	Comatose, unresponsive	___
Fractures	None	Closed (or suspected)	Multiple open or closed	___
Wounds	None	Minor**	Major,** burns, or penetrating	___
TOTAL			−6 to +12	___

Score: Possible −6 to +12, decreasing with injury severity

Generally: 9-12 → minor trauma
6-8 → potentially life threatening
0-5 → life threatening
<0 → usually fatal

*No assistance required.
†Protected by patient but constant observation required for position, patency, or O_2 administration.
‡Invasive techniques required for control (e.g., intubation).
§Responds to voice, pain, or temporary loss of consciousness.
**Abrasions or lacerations.

ADULT BURN CHART

Guidelines for rapidly estimating the percentage of body surface area burned

Note: For all ages, palms & genitalia are each ≅ 1% & buttocks ≅ 5% of total body surface area (BSA).

Severity/Degree/% Surface Area

	Degree		
Severity	**1°**	**2°**	**3°**
Minor	<20%	<15%	<2%
Moderate	>20%	>15%	>2%
Severe*		>30%	>10%

Parkland Guide to Fluid Resuscitation of Burn Patients

2-4 ml/kg/ % burn over the 1st 24 hr.
Give about ½ during the 1st 8 hr,
then the other ½ during the next 16 hr

or 0.25 × weight (kg) × % burn = ml/hr

Note: Adequate urine output is @ least 30-50 ml/hr.

*Or, associated with fractures, respiratory tract, genitalia, hands, feet, or secondary causes.

ADULT BURN CHART

"Rule of nines"

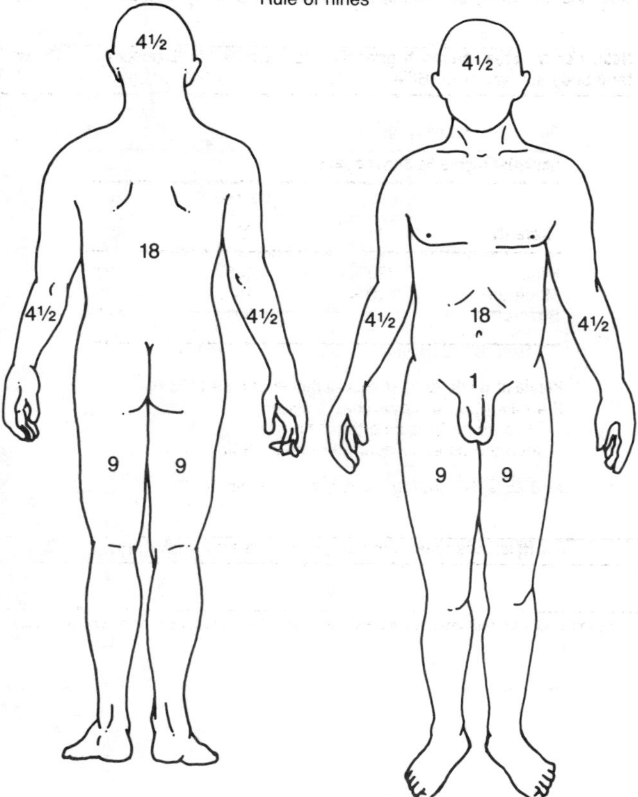

PEDIATRIC BURN CHART

Guidelines for rapidly estimating the percentage of body surface area burned

Note: For all ages, palms & genitalia are each ≅ 1% & buttocks ≅ 5% of total body surface area (BSA).

Severity/Degree/% Surface Area

	Degree		
Severity	**1°**	**2°**	**3°**
Minor	<20%	<15%	<2%
Moderate	>20%	>15%	>2%
Severe*		>30%	>10%

Parkland Guide to Fluid Resuscitation of Burn Patients
4 ml/kg/ % burn over the 1st 24 hr.
Give about ½ during the 1st 8 hr,
then the other ½ over the next 16 hr

Note: Adequate urine output is @ least 1-2 ml/kg/hr.

*Or, associated with fractures, respiratory tract, genitalia, hands, feet, or secondary causes.

PEDIATRIC BURN CHART

Child

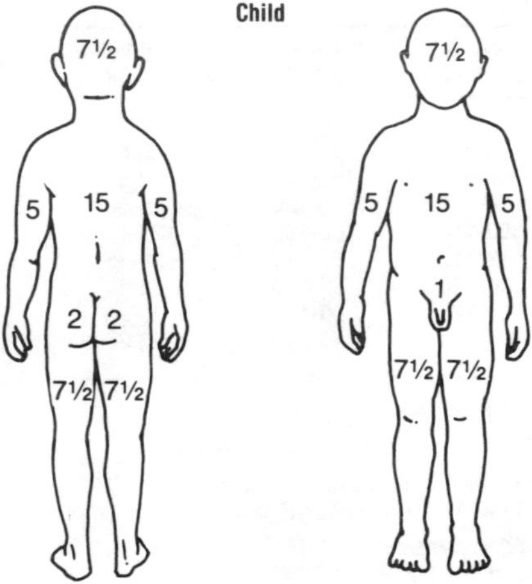

Infant

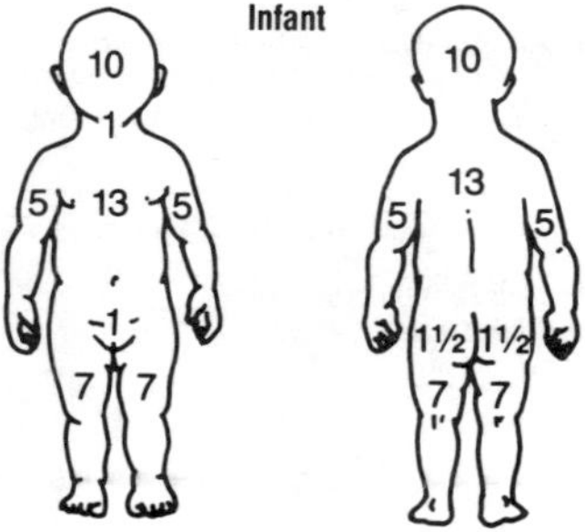

PEDIATRIC MISCELLANEOUS

Normal Vital Signs

Age	Syst. BP (mmHg)	Pulse (/min)	Respirations (/min)
Neonate	60-90	90-145	30-70
1 mo	60-90	115-190	20-60
3 mo	65-95	110-190	20-60
6 mo	74-100	110-180	20-50
1 yr	80-112	100-160	20-40
3 yr	82-115	90-150	20-35
5 yr	84-120	80-120	20-30
10 yr	84-120	60-110	15-25
13 yr	94-140	50-110	10-20

Approximate BP (for >1 yr)
80 + [2 × age (yr)]

Hypotension Estimation:
= systolic BP <70 mmHg + [2 × age (yr)]

Hypovolemic Fluid Replacement
About 10-20 ml/kg/dose over ≃ 10 min

Urine Output
1-2 ml/kg/hr is adequate

Bradycardia / CPR
Initiate CPR on neonates if pulse drops below 50-60/min

Defibrillation
Initially 2 J/kg, if unsuccessful → 4 J/kg

Cardioversion
0.5-1 J/kg

Pediatric Rule of 6 (for calculating drug dosages):
wt (kg) × 0.6 = mg added for a total volume of 100 ml &
1 ml/hr = 0.1 μg/kg/min

or

wt (kg) × 6 = mg added for a total volume of 100 ml &
1 ml/hr = 1 μg/kg/min

PEDIATRIC AGE-WEIGHT-ET-SUCTION-GASTRIC-CHEST TUBE SIZES

This table represents averages based on weight. It should be remembered that these are only *guidelines*.

Age	Weight		ET tube (mm)	Suction catheter (F)	Gastric tube (F)	Chest tube (F)
	kg	lb				
Premie	<3	<6.5	2.5-3.0	5-8	5	12
Neonate	3.5	7	3.0-3.5	6-8	5-8	
3 mo	5.0	11	3.5-4.0	6-8	8-10	
6 mo	6.5	15	3.5-4.0	8-10	8-10	16
9 mo	8.5	18	3.5-4.0	8-10	8-10	
1 yr	10.0	22	4.0-5.0	8-10	10-12	
1.5 yr	11.5	25	4.0-5.0	8-10	10-12	
2 yr	12.0	26	4.5-5.5	8-10	10-12	
3 yr	15.0	33	4.5-5.5	8-12	10-12	
4 yr	17.0	37	5.0-5.5	10-12	10-12	
5 yr	18.0	40	5.0-6.0	10-14	10-12	24
6 yr	21.5	44	5.5-6.5	10-14	10-12	
7 yr	22.5	50	6.0-6.5	10-14	10-12	
8 yr	26.0	56	6.0-6.5	10-14	10-12	28
9 yr	28.0	60	6.0-7.0	10-14	10-14	
10 yr	33.0	70	6.5-7.0	10-14	12-14	
12 yr	39.0	86	6.5-7.5	10-14	12-14	
14 yr	49.0	108	7.0-7.5	10-14	12-16	
16 yr	56.0	123	7.0-7.5	10-14	12-16	

Weight Estimation:

a. Wt (kg) = [2 × age (yr)] + 8 (from 1-9 yr)

b. Wt (kg) = 10 kg for 1st yr,
then add 2 kg for each additional yr

ETT Size Estimation:

a. $\frac{\text{Age (yr)}}{4} + 4$

b. $\frac{16 + \text{age (yr)}}{4}$ (for >1 yr)

c. Nostril or little finger diameter

APGAR SCORE

Commonly recorded at birth, 5 min, & at 10 min postdelivery

Physical sign	Points			Score
	0	**1**	**2**	
Appearance	Blue/pale	Pink body/blue extremities	All pink	___
Pulse	Absent	<100/min	>100/min	___
Grimace (reflex response irritability to suction)	None	Grimace	Cough, cry, sneeze	___
Activity (muscle tone)	Flaccid	Some flexion	Active movement	___
Respirations	Absent	Weak cry, slow irregular	Strong cry, good volume	___
TOTAL			0-10	___

Score: Possible 0-10, decreasing with severity
Generally: 7-10 → O.K.
4-6 → moderately depressed
0-3 → severely depressed

Note: Any resuscitative effort should be based on HR (pulse), respiratory activity, and color, rather than entire score.

Note: If <7, record q 5 min for a total of 20 min.

EQUIVALENTS AND CONVERSIONS

LIQUID VOLUME

Apothecary (household)	Approximate metric (ml)
1 gallon (gal)	4000
1 quart (qt)	1000
1 pint (pt)	500
1/2 pint	250
1 cup	240
1 ounce (oz)	30
1 tablespoon (tbsp)	15
1 teaspoon (tsp)	5

WEIGHTS

Apothecary (household)	Approximate metric
2.2 pounds (lb)	1 kg
1 pound	500 g
1 ounce (oz)	30 g
15 grains (gr)	1 g
1 grain	60 mg
1/60 grain	1 mg

PRESSURES

14.7 psi = 1 atm = 760 torr = 760 mmHg
1 psi = 6.9 kPa
1 kPa = 0.15 psi
1 cmH_2O = 1.36 mmHg
1 mmHg = 0.74 cmH_2O

MISCELLANEOUS

1 ml = 1 cc

IV Tubing:
1 ml = 60 microdrops
1 ml = 20, 15, or 10 macrodrops (depends on the manufacturer)
°C = (°F − 32) × 5/9
°F = (°C × 9/5) + 32
1 Joule (J) = 1 watt-second (w-s)

FORMULA—DRUG DOSAGE/IV FLOW RATE

Note: For pediatric formula, see Pediatric Miscellaneous.

DRUG DOSAGE FORMULA

(For quick calculation of drug dosages)

$$\textbf{\textit{drug volume to be administered (ml)}} = \frac{\text{desired dose (mg)}}{\text{drug concentration (mg/ml)}}$$

$$\textit{or} = \frac{\text{desired dose (mg)} \times \text{volume (ml)}}{\text{amount (mg)}}$$

> **Note:** $\text{drug concentration (mg/ml)} = \frac{\text{amount (mg)}}{\text{volume (ml)}}$

IV FLOW RATE FORMULA

$$\textbf{flow rate (ml/hr)} = \frac{\text{desired dose (mg/min)} \times 60 \text{ (min/hr)}}{\text{drug concentration (mg/ml)}}$$

$$\textbf{flow rate (ml/hr)} = \frac{\text{desired dose } (\mu\text{g/kg/min}) \times 60 \text{ (min/hr)} \times \text{wt (kg)}}{\text{drug concentration } (\mu\text{g/ml})}$$

$$\textbf{flow rate (ml/hr)} = \frac{\text{drip rate (drops/min)} \times 60 \text{ (min/hr)}}{60 \text{ (drops/ml)}}$$

$$\textbf{drip rate (drops/min)} = \frac{\text{total volume to be infused (ml)} \times \text{drop factor (drops/ml)}}{\text{total time for the infusion (min)}}$$

or

$$\textbf{drip rate (drops/min)} = \frac{\text{drops/ml}}{60 \text{ (min/hr)}} \times \frac{\text{volume to be infused (ml/hr)}}{1}$$

CONVERSIONS—DRUG DOSAGE/IV FLOW RATE

1. a. from **mg/min *to* ml/hr:**

$$\frac{\text{dose ordered (mg/min)} \times 60\ \text{(min/hr)}}{\text{concentration in bag (mg/ml)}}$$

   b. from **ml/hr *to* mg/min:**

$$\frac{\text{concentration in bag (mg/ml)} \times \text{rate (ml/hr)}}{60\ \text{(min/hr)}}$$

2. a. from **μg/min *to* ml/hr:**

$$\frac{\text{dose ordered (}\mu\text{g/min)} \times \text{(60 min/hr)}}{\text{concentration in bag (}\mu\text{g/ml)}}$$

   b. from **ml/hr *to* μg/min:**

$$\frac{\text{concentration in bag (}\mu\text{g/ml)} \times \text{rate (ml/hr)}}{60\ \text{(min/hr)}}$$

3. a. from **μg/kg/min *to* ml/hr:**

$$\frac{\text{weight (kg)} \times \text{dose ordered (}\mu\text{g/kg/min)} \times \text{(60 min/hr)}}{\text{concentration in bag (}\mu\text{g/ml)}}$$

   b. from **ml/hr *to* μg/kg/min:**

$$\frac{\text{concentration in bag (}\mu\text{g/ml)} \times \text{rate (ml/hr)} \div \text{(60 min/hr)}}{\text{weight (kg)}}$$

ADULT NORMAL LAB VALUES*

	Old	Standard international (SI)
ABGs		
pH	7.35-7.45	7.35-7.45
PCO_2	35-45 mm Hg	4.4-6.0 kPa
PO_2	80-100 mm Hg	10.0-14.0 kPa
HCO_3^-	20-28 mEq/L	20-28 mmol/L
SaO_2	>94%	>94%
BE (base excess)	±2	±2
Hematology		
Hgb male	13-18 g/100 ml	130-180 g/L
female	11-16 g/100 ml	110-160 g/L
Hct male	40-54 vol %	0.40-0.54
female	35-49 vol %	0.35-0.49
PT	10-15 sec	10-15 sec
PTT	25-70 sec	25-70 sec
RBCs male	$4.5\text{-}6.2 \times 10^6/mm^3$	$4.5\text{-}6.2 \times 10^9/L$
female	$4\text{-}5.5 \times 10^6/mm^3$	$4\text{-}5.5 \times 10^9/L$
WBCs	$5\text{-}11 \times 10^3/mm^3$	$4\text{-}11 \times 10^9/L$
PLTs	$140\text{-}500 \times 10^3/mm^3$	$140\text{-}500 \times 10^9/L$
Electrolytes		
Na^+	135-153 mEq/L	135-153 mmol/L
K^+	3.2-5.6 mEq/L	3.2-5.6 mmol/L
Cl^-	96-112 mEq/L	96-112 mmol/L
Ca^{++}	2.1-2.6 mEq/L	2.1-2.6 mmol/L
Chemistry		
BG (fasting)	60-110 mg/100 ml	2.8-6.0 mmol/L
BG (2 hr p.c.)	<120 mg/100 ml	3.9-6.1 mmol/L
Bun	7-18 mg/100 ml	1.79-8.93 mmol/L
Creatine (serum)	0.17-0.70 mg/100 ml	50-110 μmol/L
Miscellaneous		

*Normal laboratory values are subject to variation depending on individual differences in lab equipment, methods, & personnel.

Section Five

Classes of Common Home (Prescription) Drugs

INTRODUCTION TO CLASSES OF COMMON HOME (PRESCRIPTION) DRUGS

The drugs in this section are those that prehospital care personnel may encounter frequently.

Various prescription drugs may cause adverse effects in patients, especially when taken inappropriately or not taken at all. Having some knowledge of those drugs and a quick reference guide may provide you with valuable insight into the patient's presenting condition or into potential problems and will assist in planning patient care (especially in the administration of emergency drugs).

I have used a modified format of that used for the emergency drugs to provide the pertinent information on home drugs to prehospital care personnel. There are often many different drugs within the same class, and *information is therefore very general in nature* (out of necessity in a pocketbook like this).

It should be kept in mind that some drugs may have different or multiple uses depending on patient condition. For example, β-blockers may have been prescribed for hypertension and angina, or recurrent tachyarrhythmia. Some drugs may also be used in combination with others to act synergistically, or at times, antagonistically.

INDEX (CROSS-REFERENCE) CLASSES OF COMMON HOME (PRESCRIPTION) DRUGS

This index was developed to provide a quick reference to drug class/type of home prescription drugs that are commonly encountered by prehospital personnel.

1. Drugs are listed by common generic (boldface type) and by common Canadian and U.S. trade name(s) (lightface type), followed by class/type.
2. There may be more than one trade name for a given generic name.
3. Some trade name drugs are combination products (i.e., made up of two or more generic drugs, e.g., Aldactazide **Hydrochlorothiazide-Spironolactone**).
4. Some drugs may belong to more than one class/type.

> **Note:** Some of these medications may not have a corresponding classification page.

How to Use this Section

1. Look up the drug name and classification, then go to the classification page to find general information on that drug.
2. If you know the classification of the drug, go directly to the classification page.

Acebutolol Sectral: antiarrhythmic (class II)
Acenocoumarol Sintrom: anticoagulant
Acetaminophen, Paracetamol Tylenol, Tempra: analgesic, antipyretic
Acetazolamide Diamox: diuretic
Acetohexamide Dimelor: antidiabetic (oral hypoglycemic)
Acetophenazine Tindal: antipsychotic, antiemetic (phenothiazine)
Acetyldigitoxin Acylanid: cardiac glycoside (cardiotonic)
Acylanid **Acetyldigitoxin:** cardiac glycoside (cardiotonic)
Adalat **Nifedipine:** Ca^{++} channel blocker, antianginal
Adapin **Doxepin:** antidepressant (TCA)
Albuterol Proventil: bronchodilator (sympathomimetic)
Aldactazide **Hydrochlorothiazide-Spironolactone:** diuretic
Aldactone **Spironolactone:** diuretic
Aldomet **Methyldopa:** antihypertensive
Alphaprodine Nisentil: analgesic (narcotic)
Alprazolam Xanax: anxiolytic, sedative (benzodiazepine)
Alupent **Orciprenaline:** bronchodilator (sympathomimetic)
Aminophylline Phyllocontin & various: bronchodilator (theophylline)
Amiodarone Cordarone: antiarrhythmic (class III)
Amitid **Amitriptyline:** antidepressant (TCA)
Amitriptyline Elavil & various: antidepressant (TCA)
Amobarbital Amytal & various: sedative-hypnotic, anticonvulsant (barbiturate)
Amoxapine Asendin: antidepressant (TCA)
Amytal **Amobarbital:** sedative-hypnotic, anticonvulsant (barbiturate)
Anafranil **Clomipramine:** antidepressant (TCA)
Ancasal **ASA-Caffeine-Codeine:** analgesic (narcotic), antipyretic
Apresoline **Hydralazine:** antihypertensive (vasodilator)
Asendin **Amoxapine:** antidepressant (TCA)
Atarax **Hydroxyzine:** anxiolytic, antihistamine (piperazine)
Atasol **Acetaminophen-Caffeine-Codeine:** analgesic (narcotic), antipyretic
Atenol **Atenolol:** β-blocker
Atenolol Tenormin, Atenol: β-blocker
Ativan **Lorazepam:** anxiolytic, sedative (benzodiazepine)
Atrovent **Ipratropium:** bronchodilator
Aventyl **Nortriptyline:** antidepressant (TCA)
Beclomethasone Beclovent, Vanceril: bronchodilator (steroid)
Beclovent **Beclomethasone:** bronchodilator (steroid)
Benzphetamine Didrex: CNS stimulant (amphetamine)
Berotec **Fenoterol:** bronchodilator (sympathomimetic)
Betaloc **Metoprolol:** β-blocker, antihypertensive, antianginal
Biquin **Quinidine:** antiarrhythmic (class Ia)
Bitolterol Tornalate: bronchodilator (sympathomimetic)

Blocadren **Timolol:** β-blocker, antianginal, antihypertensive
Brethaire **Terbutaline:** bronchodilator (sympathomimetic)
Brethine **Terbutaline:** bronchodilator (sympathomimetic)
Bricanyl **Terbutaline:** bronchodilator (sympathomimetic)
Bromazepam Lectopam: anxiolytic, sedative (benzodiazepine)
Bronkaid **Epinephrine:** bronchodilator (sympathomimetic)
Bronkometer **Isoetharine:** bronchodilator (sympathomimetic)
Bronkosol **Isoetharine:** bronchodilator (sympathomimetic)
Butabarbital Butisol, Day-Barb, Mebutal: sedative-hypnotic (barbiturate)
Butisol **Butabarbital:** sedative-hypnotic (barbiturate)
Calan **Verapamil:** Ca^{++} channel blocker, antianginal, antiarrhythmic
Capoten **Captopril:** antihypertensive
Captopril Capoten: antihypertensive
Carbamazepine Tegretol: anticonvulsant
Cardilate **Erythrityl Tetranitrate:** antianginal (coronary vasodilator)
Cardizem **Diltiazem:** Ca^{++} channel blocker, antianginal
Catapres **Clonidine:** antihypertensive
Cedilanid **Deslanoside:** cardiac glycoside (cardiotonic)
Celontin **Methsuximide:** anticonvulsant (succinimide)
Centrax **Prazepam:** sedative-hypnotic, antianxiety (benzodiazepine)
Chloral Hydrate Noctec: sedative-hypnotic
Chlordiazepoxide Librium & various: antianxiety (benzodiazepine)
Chlorothiazide Diuril: diuretic
Chlorpromazine Largactil, Thorazine: antipsychotic, antiemetic (phenothiazine)
Chlorpropamide Diabinese: antidiabetic (oral hypoglycemic)
Chlorprothixene Tarasan, Tartactan: antipsychotic, antiemetic (phenothiazine)
Chlorthalidone Uridon, Igroton: diuretic, antihypertensive
Choledyl **Oxtriphylline:** bronchodilator (theophylline)
Clomipramine Anafranil: antidepressant (TCA)
Clonazepam Rivotril, Klonopin: anticonvulsant (benzodiazepine)
Clonidine Catapres: antihypertensive
Clorazepate Tranxene: anxiolytic, sedative, anticonvulsant (benzodiazepine)
Codeine, Methylmorphine: analgesic (narcotic), antitussive
Combipres **Clonidine-Chlorthalidone:** antihypertensive
Cordarone **Amiodarone:** antiarrhythmic (class III)
Corgard **Nadolol:** β-blocker, antianginal, antihypertensive
Coronex **Isosorbide:** antianginal (coronary vasodilator)
Coumadin **Warfarin:** anticoagulant
Crystodigin **Digitoxin:** cardiac glycoside (cardiotonic)
Dalmane **Flurazepam:** hypnotic (benzodiazepine)
Darvocet **Propoxyphene-Acetaminophen:** analgesic (narcotic)

Darvon **Propoxyphene:** analgesic (narcotic)
Day-Barb **Butabarbital:** sedative-hypnotic (barbiturate)
Demerol **Meperidine:** analgesic (narcotic)
Depakene **Valproic Acid:** anticonvulsant (uncategorized)
Depakote **Divalproex:** anticonvulsant
Desipramine Norpramin, Pertofrane: antidepressant (TCA)
Deslanoside Cedilanid: cardiac glycoside (cardiotonic)
Desyrel **Trazodone:** antidepressant (miscellaneous)
Detensol **Propranolol:** β-blocker, antianginal, antihypertensive, antiarrhythmic
Dexamphetamine Dexedrine, Synatan: CNS stimulant (sympathomimetic)
Dexedrine **Dexamphetamine:** CNS stimulant (sympathomimetic)
Dextromethorphan (various cough syrups): expectorant (narcotic)
Diaβeta **Glyburide:** antidiabetic (oral hypoglycemic)
Diabinese **Chlorpropamide:** antidiabetic (oral hypoglycemic)
Diamox **Acetazolamide:** diuretic
Diazepam Valium, Vivol: anxiolytic, sedative, muscle relaxant (benzodiazepine)
Dicoumarin see **Dicumarol**
Dicumarol Dicumin: anticoagulant
Dicumin **Dicumarol:** anticoagulant
Didrex **Benzphetamine:** CNS stimulant (amphetamine)
Digitaline **Digitoxin:** cardiac glycoside (cardiotonic)
Digitoxin Digitaline, Crystodigin: cardiac glycoside (cardiotonic)
Digoxin Lanoxin: cardiac glycoside (cardiotonic)
Dilantin **Phenytoin:** anticonvulsant (hydantoin), antiarrhythmic (class Ib)
Dilaudid **Hydromorphone:** analgesic (narcotic)
Diltiazem Cardizem, Tilazem: Ca^{++} channel blocker, antianginal
Dimelor **Acetohexamide:** antidiabetic (oral hypoglycemic)
Diphenhydramine Benadryl: antihistamine
Dipyridamole Persantine: antianginal (coronary vasodilator, platelet inhibitor)
Disopyramide Rhythmodan, Norpace: antiarrhythmic (class Ia)
Diuril **Chlorothiazide:** diuretic
Divalproex Epival, Depakote: anticonvulsant
Dolophine **Methadone:** analgesic (narcotic)
Donnatal **Belladonna-Phenobarbital:** sedative, antispasmodic
Doriden **Glutethimide:** sedative-hypnotic (piperidine)
Doxepin Sinequan, Adapin: antidepressant (TCA)
Duretic **Methyclothiazide:** diuretic
Dyazide **Hydrochlorothiazide-Triamterene:** diuretic, antihypertensive
Dyrenium **Triamterene:** diuretic
Edecrin **Ethacrynic Acid:** diuretic
Elavil **Amitriptyline:** antidepressant (TCA)

Empracet **Acetaminophen-Codeine:** analgesic (narcotic), antipyretic, antitussive
Emtec **Acetaminophen-Codeine:** analgesic (narcotic), antipyretic, antitussive
Endep **Amitriptyline:** antidepressant (TCA)
Enduron **Methyclothiazide:** diuretic
Epimorph **Morphine:** analgesic (narcotic)
Epinephrine Bronkaid, Micronefrin, Vaponefrin: bronchodilator (sympathomimetic)
Epival **Divalproex:** anticonvulsant
Equanil **Meprobamate:** antianxiety (carbamate)
Esidrix **Hydrochlorothiazide:** diuretic, antihypertensive
Ethacrynic Acid Edecrin: diuretic
Ethchlorvynol Placidyl: sedative-hypnotic (uncategorized)
Ethosuximide Zarontin: anticonvulsant (succinimide)
Etrafon **Amitriptyline-Perphenazine:** antidepressant (TCA), antipsychotic (phenothiazine)
Euglucon **Glyburide:** antidiabetic (oral hypoglycemic)
Eutonyl **Pargyline:** antidepressant (MAOI)
Exdol **Acetaminophen-Caffeine-Codeine:** analgesic (narcotic), antipyretic
Fentoterol Berotec: bronchodilator (sympathomimetic)
Fivent **Sodium Cromoglycate:** bronchodilator (uncategorized)
Flecanide Tambocor: antiarrhythmic (class Ic)
Fluphenazine Permitil, Prolixin, & various: antipsychotic (phenothiazine)
Flupromazine Vesprin: antipsychotic (phenothiazine)
Flurazepam Dalmane: hypnotic (benzodiazepine)
Furosemide Lasix: diuretic
Glipizide Glucotrol: antidiabetic (oral hypoglycemic)
Glucotrol **Glipizide:** antidiabetic (oral hypoglycemic)
Glutethimide Doriden: sedative-hypnotic (piperidine)
Glyburide Diaβeta, Euglucon, Micronase: antidiabetic (oral hypoglycemic)
Guanabenz Wytensin: antihypertensive
Guanethidine Ismelin: antihypertensive
Halazepam Paxipam: sedative-hypnotic, antianxiety (benzodiazepine)
Halcion **Triazolam:** hypnotic (benzodiazepine)
Haldol **Haloperidol:** antipsychotic, antiemetic (butyrophenone)
Haloperidol Haldol, Peridol: antipsychotic, antiemetic (butyrophenone)
Hepalean **Heparin:** anticoagulant
Heparin Hepalean, Minihep: anticoagulant
Humulin **Insulin:** antidiabetic (insulin)
Hycodan **Hydrocodone:** analgesic (narcotic)
Hydralazine Apresoline: antihypertensive (vasodilator)
Hydrochlorothiazide HydroDiuril & various: diuretic, antihypertensive

Hydrocodone Hycodan: analgesic (narcotic)
HydroDiuril **Hydrochlorothiazide:** diuretic, antihypertensive
Hydromorphone Dilaudid: analgesic (narcotic)
Hydropres **Hydrochlorothiazide-Reserpine:** diuretic, antihypertensive
Hydroxyzine Atarax, Vistaril: anxiolytic, antihistamine (piperazine)
Igroton **Chlorthalidone:** diuretic, antihypertensive
Iletin **Insulin:** antidiabetic (insulin)
Imavate **Imipramine:** antidepressant (TCA)
Imipramine Tofranil & various: antidepressant (TCA)
Inderal **Propranolol:** β-blocker, antianginal, antihypertensive, antiarrhythmic
Inderide **Propranolol-Hydrochlorothiazide:** antihypertensive
Insulin (various): antidiabetic (insulin)
Intal **Sodium Cromoglycate:** bronchodilator (uncategorized)
Ipratropium Atrovent: bronchodilator
Ismelin **Guanethidine:** antihypertensive
Isocarboxazid Marplan: antidepressant (MAOI)
Isoetharine Bronkosol: bronchodilator (sympathomimetic)
Isoptin **Verapamil:** Ca^{++} channel blocker, antianginal, antiarrhythmic
Isordil **Isosorbide:** antianginal (coronary vasodilator)
Isosorbide Isordil: antianginal (coronary vasodilator)
Ketazolam Loftran: anxiolytic, sedative (benzodiazepine)
Klonopin **Clonazepam:** anticonvulsant (benzodiazepine)
Labetolol Trandate: β-blocker, antiarrhythmic (class Ic)
Lanoxin **Digoxin:** cardiac glycoside (cardiotonic)
Largactil **Chlorpromazine:** antipsychotic, antiemetic (phenothiazine)
Lasix **Furosemide:** diuretic
Lectopam **Bromazepam:** anxiolytic, sedative (benzodiazepine)
Librium **Chlordiazepoxide:** antianxiety (benzodiazepine)
Lidocaine LidoPen: antiarrhythmic (class Ib)
Limbitrol **Chlordiazepoxide-Amitriptyline:** antianxiety (benzodiazepine)-antidepressant (TCA)
Lithane **Lithium:** antipsychotic (alkali metal salt)
Lithium Lithane & various: antipsychotic (alkali metal salt)
Lithizine **Lithium:** antipsychotic (alkali metal salt)
Loftran **Ketazolam:** anxiolytic, sedative (benzodiazepine)
Loniten **Minoxidil:** antihypertensive
Lopressor **Metoprolol:** β-blocker, antianginal, antihypertensive
Lorazepam Ativan: anxiolytic, sedative (benzodiazepine)
Ludiomil **Maprotiline:** antidepressant (TCA)
Luminal **Phenobarbital:** sedative, anticonvulsant (barbiturate)
Mandrax **Methaqualone-Diphenhydramine:** hypnotic
Maprotiline Ludiomil: antidepressant (TCA)

Marplan **Isocarboxazid:** antidepressant (MAOI)
Mebaral **Mephobarbital:** sedative, anticonvulsant (barbiturate)
Mebroin **Mephobarbital-Phenytoin:** antiepileptic (barbiturate-hydantoin)
Mebutal **Butabarbital:** sedative-hypnotic (barbiturate)
Medihaler-Epi **Epinephrine:** bronchodilator (sympathomimetic)
Mellaril **Thioridazine:** antipsychotic, tranquilizer (phenothiazine)
Meperidine Demerol: analgesic (narcotic)
Mephenytoin Mesantoin: anticonvulsant (hydantoin)
Mephobarbital Mebaral: sedative, anticonvulsant (barbiturate)
Meprobamate Miltown, Equanil: antianxiety (carbamate)
Mesantoin **Mephenytoin:** anticonvulsant (hydantoin)
Mesoridazine Serentil: antipsychotic (phenothiazine)
Metaprel **Metaproterenol:** bronchodilator (sympathomimetic)
Metaproterenol Metaprel: bronchodilator (sympathomimetic)
Methadone Dolophine: analgesic (narcotic)
Methaqualone Quaalude: sedative-hypnotic
Methotrimeprazine Nozinan: antipsychotic, analgesic (phenothiazine)
Methsuximide Celontin: anticonvulsant (succinimide)
Methyclothiazide Duretic, Enduron: diuretic
Methyldopa Aldomet: antihypertensive
Methylmorphine see **Codeine**
Methylphenidate Ritalin: CNS stimulant (piperidine)
Methyprylon Noludar: hypnotic (piperidine)
Metoprolol Lopressor, Betaloc: β-blocker, antihypertensive, antianginal
Mexiletine Mexitil: antiarrhythmic (class Ib)
Mexitil **Mexiletine:** antiarrhythmic (class Ib)
Micronase **Glyburide:** antidiabetic (oral hypoglycemic)
Micronefrin **Epinephrine:** bronchodilator (sympathomimetic)
Milontin **Phensuximide:** anticonvulsant (succinimide)
Miltown **Meprobamate:** anxiolytic, sedative-hypnotic (carbamate)
Minihep **Heparin:** anticoagulant
Minipress **Prazosin:** antihypertensive
Minoxidil Loniten: antihypertensive
Mobenol **Tolbutamide:** antidiabetic (oral hypoglycemic)
Moduret **Hydrochlorothiazide-Amiloride:** diuretic, antihypertensive
Mogadon **Nitrazepam:** hypnotic, anticonvulsant (benzodiazepine)
Morphine Epimorph: analgesic (narcotic)
Multipax **Hydroxyzine:** anxiolytic, antihistamine
Mysoline **Primidone:** anticonvulsant ("non-barbiturate")
Nadolol Corgard: β-blocker, antianginal, antihypertensive
Nardil **Phenelzine:** antidepressant (MAOI)
Navane **Thiothixene:** antipsychotic (thioxanthene)

Nembutal **Pentobarbital:** sedative-hypnotic (barbiturate)
Nifedipine Adalat, Procardia: Ca^{++} channel blocker, antianginal
Nisentil **Alphaprodine:** analgesic (narcotic)
Nitrazepam Mogadon: hypnotic, anticonvulsant (benzodiazepine)
Nitrobid **Nitroglycerin:** antianginal (coronary vasodilator)
Nitrogard **Nitroglycerin:** antianginal (coronary vasodilator)
Nitroglycerin (various): antianginal (coronary vasodilator)
Nitrol **Nitroglycerin:** antianginal (coronary vasodilator)
Nitrolingual **Nitroglycerin:** antianginal (coronary vasodilator)
Nitrong **Nitroglycerin:** antianginal (coronary vasodilator)
Nitrostabilin **Nitroglycerin:** antianginal (coronary vasodilator)
Nitrostat **Nitroglycerin:** antianginal (coronary vasodilator)
Noctec **Chloral Hydrate:** sedative-hypnotic
Noludar **Methyprylon:** hypnotic (piperidine)
Norpace **Disopyramide:** antiarrhythmic (class Ia)
Norpramin **Desipramine:** antidepressant (TCA)
Nortriptyline Aventyl, Pamelor: antidepressant (TCA)
Novolin **Insulin:** antidiabetic (insulin)
Nozinan **Methotrimeprazine:** antipsychotic, analgesic (phenothiazine)
Numorphan **Oxymorphone:** analgesic (narcotic)
Orciprenaline Alupent: bronchodilator (sympathomimetic)
Orinase **Tolbutamide:** antidiabetic (oral hypoglycemic)
Oxazepam Serax: antianxiety (benzodiazepine)
Oxprenolol Trasicor: β-blocker
Oxtriphylline Choledyl: bronchodilator (theophylline)
Oxycocet **Oxycodone-Acetaminophen:** analgesic (narcotic)
Oxycodan **Oxycodone-ASA:** analgesic (narcotic)
Oxymorphone Numorphan: analgesic (narcotic)
Pamelor **Nortriptyline:** antidepressant (TCA)
Paracetamol see **Acetaminophen**
Paregoric **Opium tincture:** antidiarrheal (narcotic)
Parepectolin **Opium-Kaolin-Pectin:** antidiarrheal (narcotic)
Pargyline Eutonyl: antidepressant (MAOI)
Parnate **Tranylcypromine:** antidepressant (MAOI)
Paxipam **Halazepam:** sedative-hypnotic, antianxiety (benzodiazepine)
PBR/12 **Phenobarbital:** sedative-hypnotic, anticonvulsant (barbiturate)
Pentazocine Talwin: analgesic (narcotic)
Pentobarbital Nembutal: sedative-hypnotic (barbiturate)
Percocet **Oxycodone-Acetaminophen:** analgesic (narcotic)
Percodan: **Oxycodone-ASA:** analgesic (narcotic)
Peridol **Haloperidol:** antipsychotic, antiemetic (butyrophenone)
Permitil **Fluphenazine:** antipsychotic (phenothiazine)

Perphenazine Trilafon: antipsychotic, antiemetic (phenothiazine)
Persantine **Dipyridamole:** antianginal (coronary vasodilator, platelet inhibitor)
Pertofrane **Desipramine:** antidepressant (TCA)
Phenelzine Nardil: antidepressant (MAOI)
Phenobarbital Luminal: sedative, anticonvulsant (barbiturate)
Phensuximide Milontin: anticonvulsant (succinimide)
Phenytoin Dilantin: anticonvulsant (hydantoin), antiarrhythmic (class Ib)
Phyllocontin **Aminophylline:** bronchodilator (theophylline)
Pindolol Visken: β-blocker, antihypertensive, antianginal
Piperacetazine Quide: antipsychotic (phenothiazine)
Placidyl **Ethchlorvynol:** sedative-hypnotic (uncategorized)
Prazepam Centrax: sedative-hypnotic, antianxiety (benzodiazepine)
Prazosin Minipress: antihypertensive
Presamine **Imipramine:** antidepressant (TCA)
Primidone Mysoline: anticonvulsant ("non-barbiturate")
Procainamide Pronestyl, Procan: antiarrhythmic (class Ia)
Procan **Procainamide:** antiarrhythmic (class Ia)
Procardia **Nifedipine:** Ca^{++} channel blocker, antianginal
Prochlorperazine Stemetil: antipsychotic, antiemetic (phenothiazine)
Prolixin **Fluphenazine:** antipsychotic (phenothiazine)
Promazine Sparine: antipsychotic, antiemetic (phenothiazine)
Pronestyl **Procainamide:** antiarrhythmic (class Ia)
Propoxyphene Darvon: analgesic (narcotic)
Propranolol Inderal, Detensol: β-blocker, antianginal, antihypertensive, antiarrhythmic
Prosedyl **Quinidine:** antiarrhythmic (class Ia)
Protriptyline Triptil, Vivactil: antidepressant (TCA)
Proventil **Albuterol:** bronchodilator (sympathomimetic)
Quaalude **Methaqualone:** sedative-hypnotic
Quibron **Theophylline:** bronchodilator (theophylline)
Quide **Piperacetazine:** antipsychotic (phenothiazine)
Quinaglute **Quinidine:** antiarrhythmic (class Ia)
Quinate **Quinidine:** antiarrhythmic (class Ia)
Quinidex **Quinidine:** antiarrhythmic (class Ia)
Quinidine (various): antiarrhythmic (class Ia)
Quinine **Quinidine:** antiarrhythmic (class Ia)
Reserpine Serpasil: antihypertensive, antipsychotic
Restoril **Temazepam:** hypnotic (benzodiazepine)
Rhythmodan **Disopyramide:** antiarrhythmic (class Ia)
Ritalin **Methylphenidate:** CNS stimulant (piperidine)
Rivotril **Clonazepam:** anticonvulsant (benzodiazepine)
Salbutamol Ventolin: bronchodilator (sympathomimetic)

Secobarbital Seconal: sedative-hypnotic (barbiturate)
Seconal **Secobarbital:** sedative-hypnotic (barbiturate)
Sectral **Acebutolol:** antiarrhythmic (class II)
Serax **Oxazepam:** anxiolytic-sedative (benzodiazepine)
Serentil **Mesoridazine:** antipsychotic (phenothiazine)
Serpasil **Reserpine:** antihypertensive, antipsychotic
Sinequan **Doxepin:** antidepressant (TCA)
Sintrom **Acenocoumarol:** anticoagulant
Somophylline **Theophylline:** bronchodilator (theophylline)
Sotacor **Sotalol:** β-blocker, antianginal, antihypertensive
Sotalol Sotacor: β-blocker, antianginal, antihypertensive, antiarrhythmic (class III)
Sparine **Promazine:** antipsychotic, antiemetic (phenothiazine)
Spironolactone Aldactone: diuretic
Stelazine **Trifluoperazine:** antipsychotic, antiemetic (phenothiazine)
Stemetil **Prochlorperazine:** antipsychotic, antiemetic (phenothiazine)
Surmontil **Trimipramine:** antidepressant (TCA)
Synatan **Dexamphetamine:** CNS stimulant (sympathomimetic)
Talwin **Pentazocine:** analgesic (narcotic)
Tambocor **Flecanide:** antiarrhythmic (class Ic)
Tarasan **Chlorprothixene:** antipsychotic, antiemetic (phenothiazine)
Tartactan **Chlorprothixene:** antipsychotic, antiemetic (phenothiazine)
Tedral **Theophylline-Ephedrine-Phenobarbital:** bronchodilator
Tegretol **Carbamazepine:** anticonvulsant
Temazepam Restoril: hypnotic (benzodiazepine)
Tempra **Acetaminophen:** antipyretic, analgesic
Tenormin **Atenolol:** β-blocker, antihypertensive, antianginal
Terbutaline Bricanyl, Brethine: bronchodilator (sympathomimetic)
Theo-Dur **Theophylline:** bronchodilator (theophylline)
Theophylline Theo-Dur & various: bronchodilator (theophylline)
Thioridazine Mellaril: antipsychotic, tranquilizer (phenothiazine)
Thiothixene Navane: antipsychotic (thioxanthene)
Thorazine **Chlorpromazine:** antipsychotic, antiemetic (phenothiazine)
Tilazem **Diltiazem:** Ca^{++} channel blocker, antianginal
Timolol Blocadren: β-blocker, antianginal, antihypertensive
Tindal **Acetophenazine:** antipsychotic (phenothiazine)
Tocainide Tonocard: antiarrhythmic (class Ib)
Tofranil **Imipramine:** antidepressant (TCA)
Tolazamide Tolinase: antidiabetic (oral hypoglycemic)
Tolbutamide Mobenol, Orinase: antidiabetic (oral hypoglycemic)
Tolinase **Tolazamide:** antidiabetic (oral hypoglycemic)
Tonocard **Tocainide:** antiarrhythmic (class Ib)

Tornalate **Bitolterol:** bronchodilator (sympathomimetic)
Trandate **Labetalol:** β-blocker, antihypertensive
Tranxene **Clorazepate:** anxiolytic, sedative, anticonvulsant (benzodiazepine)
Tranylcypromine Parnate: antidepressant (MAOI)
Trasicor **Oxprenolol:** β-blocker
Trazodone Desyrel: antidepressant (miscellaneous)
Triadapin **Doxepin:** antidepressant (TCA)
Triamterene Dyrenium: diuretic
Triavil **Amitriptyline-Perphenazine:** antidepressant (TCA), antipsychotic (phenothiazine)
Triazolam Halcion: hypnotic (benzodiazepine)
Tridione **Trimethadione:** anticonvulsant (miscellaneous)
Trifluoperazine Stelazine: antipsychotic, antiemetic (phenothiazine)
Trilafon **Perphenazine:** antipsychotic, antiemetic (phenothiazine)
Trimethadione Tridione: anticonvulsant (miscellaneous)
Trimipramine Surmontil: antidepressant (TCA)
Triptil **Protriptyline:** antidepressant (TCA)
Tuinal **Amobarbital-Secobarbital:** hypnotic (barbiturate)
Tylenol **Acetaminophen (Caffeine-Codeine):** analgesic (narcotic), antipyretic, antitussive
Tylox **Acetaminophen-Oxycodone:** analgesic (narcotic)
Uridon **Chlorthalidone:** diuretic, antihypertensive
Valium **Diazepam:** anxiolytic, sedative, muscle relaxant (benzodiazepine)
Valproic Acid Depakene: anticonvulsant (uncategorized)
Vanceril **Beclomethasone:** bronchodilator (steroid)
Vaponefrin **Epinephrine:** bronchodilator (sympathomimetic)
Velosulin **Insulin:** antidiabetic (insulin)
Ventolin **Salbutamol, Albuterol:** bronchodilator (sympathomimetic)
Verapamil Isoptin, Calan: Ca^{++} channel blocker, antianginal, antiarrhythmic
Vesprin **Flupromazine:** antipsychotic (phenothiazine)
Vicodin **Hydrocodone-Acetaminophen:** analgesic (narcotic)
Viskazide **Pindolol-Hydrochlorothiazide:** antihypertensive
Visken **Pindolol:** β-blocker, antihypertensive, antianginal
Vistaril **Hydroxyzine:** anxiolytic, antihistamine (piperazine)
Vivactil **Protriptyline:** antidepressant (TCA)
Vivol **Diazepam:** anxiolytic, sedative, muscle relaxant (benzodiazepine)
Warfarin Coumadin, Warfilone: anticoagulant
Warfilone **Warfarin:** anticoagulant
Wygesic **Propoxyphene-Acetaminophen:** analgesic (narcotic)
Wytensin **Guanabenz:** antihypertensive
Xanax **Alprazolam:** anxiolytic, sedative (benzodiazepine)
Zarontin **Ethosuximide:** anticonvulsant (succinimide)

FORMAT OF COMMON HOME (PRESCRIPTION) DRUG INFORMATION

Information for the most part pertains to immediate prehospital emergencies. Some of these classifications cover a broad range of drugs. The *information provided is very general,* out of necessity in a pocketbook.

Classification/Type

TYPE(S):	**Therapeutic Classification**
ACTIONS:	The major mechanism(s) of action & how the drug exerts its therapeutic effects.
USES:	Condition(s) for which the drugs are commonly prescribed.
ADVERSE EFFECTS:	Any effect other than those that were therapeutically intended. Usually undesirable, specific, & predictable. Often a result of too much of the drug. May include any combination of those listed. Boldface type generally indicates effects that are more common or life-threatening.
INTERACTIONS:	Presence of another drug(s) may alter the effects of either drug or promote entirely different effects.
PREPARATIONS:	Most common forms of the drug.
SPECIAL:	Miscellaneous relevant or nice-to-know information.
COMMON EXAMPLES:	Provides a few examples (listed by trade name) of drugs in this class. When given, generic names are indicated by boldface type.

TYPE(S): **Narcotic (Opiate) (natural, semisynthetic, synthetic)**

ACTIONS:

1. Analgesia (increases pain threshold)
2. Decreases anxiety, apprehension, fear
3. CNS depressant → sedation
4. Cardiovascular (decreased anxiety reduces catecholamine release; vasodilation reduces preload)

USES:

1. Pain relief
2. Cough suppression
3. Sedation for anxiety, apprehension, fear
4. Antidiarrheal

ADVERSE EFFECTS:

CVS
- **Hypotension,** bradycardia, flushing, sweating, pulmonary edema (noncardiogenic)

CNS
- **Respiratory depression, apnea, CNS depression**
- Euphoria, drowsiness, dizziness, weakness, excessive sedation, apathy
- Paradoxical CNS stimulation, nervousness, anxiety, headache, seizure, coma
- Hallucinations, delusions, mood change

Other
- **N/v, urine retention**
- May constrict or dilate pupils; may suppress cough or corneal reflex

INTERACTIONS: CNS depressants, TCAs, MAOIs: potentiate effects

PREPARATIONS: Tablet, capsule, caplet, elixir, suppository, IV

SPECIAL:

1. Narcotics have the potential for patient tolerance, abuse, & addiction
2. A withdrawal syndrome may result from abrupt cessation after chronic use

COMMON EXAMPLES:

Ancasal	**Morphine**
Atasol	Numorphan
Codeine	Oxycocet
Darvon	Oxycodan
Demerol	Percocet
Dilaudid	Percodan
Empracet	Talwin
Exdol	Tylenol with Codeine (No. 1, 2, 3, 4)

Antianginals

TYPE(S): **Nitrates & Nitrites (primarily) (also see Beta Blockers & Calcium Channel Blockers)**

ACTIONS: Nitrates & Nitrites (coronary vasodilators):

1. Vasodilation
2. Decreases myocardial work & reduces MVO_2:
   a. Reducing preload & afterload
   b. Improving coronary perfusion (including collateral)
3. May relieve coronary vasospasm

> **Note:** Nitrates & nitrites have the same pharmacological effects but differ primarily in onset, duration, potency, & route of administration.

USES:

1. Angina, AMI, CHF, post-MI
2. Coronary artery spasm, SVTs
3. To increase exercise tolerance

ADVERSE EFFECTS:

CVS
- □ **Hypotension,** bradycardia, paradoxical angina, flushing, feeling of warmth, syncope
- □ **Reflex tachycardia, palpitation**
- □ Possible reperfusion arrhythmias (via relief of coronary vasospasm)

CNS
- □ Transient or persistent **headache, dizziness,** weakness, anxiety

Other
- □ N/v, may cause slight SL burning sensation

INTERACTIONS: Hypotensives, ETOH: may potentiate hypotension

PREPARATIONS: Tablet, ointment/paste, aerosol

SPECIAL:

1. These patients usually have coronary artery disease
2. Tablets may lose potency within a few months
3. Aerosols maintain potency for up to 3 years
4. Tolerance & dependence may develop after prolonged use
5. Avoid (prolonged) contact with "Nitro" paste (e.g., during chest compression). It will be absorbed through your skin

COMMON EXAMPLES:

Cardilate	Nitrol
Coronex	Nitrolingual Spray
Isordil	Nitrong
Nitrobid	Nitrostablin
Nitrogard	Nitrostat

(Anxiolytic) Antianxiety

TYPE(S): **Primarily Benzodiazepines (minor tranquilizers)**
Also Carbamates

ACTIONS:
1. CNS depressant → sedation
2. Skeletal muscle relaxation

USES:
1. Excessive anxiety & tension (acute or chronic):
   a. Stresses of everyday life
   b. Emotional & physical disorders
   c. Tension from insomnia
2. Anticonvulsant
3. Muscle spasms
4. Adjunctive management of acute ETOH or opiate withdrawal

ADVERSE EFFECTS:[103]

CVS
- □ **Hypotension,** tachycardia

CNS
- □ **Respiratory depression, apnea,** excessive CNS depression/sedation, coma
- □ **Drowsiness, dizziness,** vertigo, **confusion, ataxia,** slurred speech, headache, amnesia, **fatigue,** weakness
- □ Occasional paradoxical irritability, excitability, aggression
- □ Hallucinations, delirium

Other
- □ N/v, pupil dilation

INTERACTIONS: CNS depressants, including ETOH: potentiate effects

PREPARATIONS: Tablet, capsule, caplet

SPECIAL:
1. These are probably the most widely prescribed class of drugs in the world
2. There is potential for tolerance, abuse, & addiction
3. A withdrawal syndrome may result from abrupt cessation after chronic use

[103]Fatalities from Benzodiazepine OD alone are rare. There is usually something else involved (e.g., ETOH) as well.

COMMON EXAMPLES:	Atarax	Multipax
	Ativan	Serax
	Donnatal	Stelazine
	Lectopam	Tranxene
	Librium	Valium
	Loftran	Vivol
	Mellaril	Xanax

Antiarrhythmics[104]

TYPE(S): **Various (classes I-IV)**

ACTIONS: Various, depends on specific antiarrhythmic:

1. (−) chronotropy
2. (+) or (−) inotropy
3. (−) dromotropy
4. Depresses automaticity
5. Reduces MVO_2
6. Suppresses PVCs
7. Suppresses reentry activity
8. Vagolytic
9. May elevate the threshold for VF

USES:

1. To maintain NSR (or a controlled/stable abnormal rhythm)
2. Prevention of chronic rhythm disturbances

ADVERSE EFFECTS:

CVS
- □ Arrhythmia, conduction disturbances, hypotension
- □ Myocardial depression, may induce/exacerbate CHF/ pulmonary edema, may precipitate angina

CNS
- □ Headache, CNS depression, altered LOC

Other
- □ N/v

INTERACTIONS: Other antiarrhythmics: may potentiate or depress effects

PREPARATIONS: Tablet, capsule

---

[104]There are many types of antiarrhythmics. Some exert primarily ventricular or supraventricular effects, whereas some act on both. Specific information is beyond the scope of this pocketbook.

SPECIAL: Usually prescribed after some type of cardiac insult

Antiarrhythmics may be classified by their predominant electrophysiologic effects (e.g., Vaughn-Williams-Singh Classification).

Class I:
Biquin
Dilantin
Mexitil
Norpace
Procan
Pronestyl
Prosedyl
Quinate
Quinidex
Quinine
Rhythmodan
Tonocard
Xylocaine

Class II:
Primarily β-blockers:
Betaloc
Blocadren
Corgard
Inderal
Lopressor
Sotacor
Tenormin
Visken

Class III:
Bretylate
Bretylol
Cordarone

Class IV:
Ca^{++} channel blockers:
Adalat
Cardizem
Isoptin
Cardiac glycosides:
Cedilanid
Crystodigin
Digitaline
Lanoxin
Novodigoxin

Anticoagulants

TYPE(S): **Warfarin or Coumarin derivatives**

ACTIONS: Decreases the ability of blood to clot:
1. Prevents further extension of the clot
2. Prolongs blood-clotting time
3. May prevent clotting

USES: Prophylaxis/Tx of blood clotting:
1. Venous thrombosis, pulmonary embolism
2. Adjunct in the Tx of coronary occlusion & TIAs
3. Home dialysis
4. Recurrent problems with blood clots
5. Tx of embolization in A-fib
6. Postthrombolytic therapy

ADVERSE EFFECTS:
- □ **Hemorrhage** (from any organ or tissue)
- □ Excessive bleeding from minor cuts, menstruation, nose bleed
- □ Melena, petechiae
- □ N/v/d

INTERACTIONS: Salicylates, some antibiotics: may prolong clotting time & increase risk of hemorrhage

PREPARATIONS: Tablet

SPECIAL:
1. Also known as "blood thinners"
2. Patients on home dialysis may take IV Heparin
3. Anti-platelet (e.g., ASA, Persantine) effects are similar to anticoagulant effects

COMMON EXAMPLES:
Coumadin
Hepalean
Heparin
Minihep
Sintrom
Warfilone

TYPE(S): **Benzodiazepines, Barbiturates, Hydantoins, Succinimides**

ACTIONS:
1. Prevents & suppresses the spread of seizure activity in the motor cortex
2. Elevates seizure threshold
3. Skeletal muscle relaxation

USES:
1. Epilepsy
2. Chronic seizures
3. Generalized tonic-clonic (grand mal) seizures
4. Absence spells (petit mal seizures)
5. Focal, Jacksonian, psychomotor, or myoclonic seizures

ADVERSE EFFECTS:

CVS
- □ Hypotension, arrhythmia

CNS
- □ **Respiratory depression/apnea**
- □ Excessive CNS depression, **ataxia, dizziness, drowsiness,** fatigue, weakness, **confusion,** behavioral disturbances, sedation, coma, amnesia
- □ Irritability, nervousness, headache
- □ Tremor, paradoxical seizure (from OD)

Other
- □ N/v/d, anorexia, abdominal pain, indigestion, constipation
- □ Visual disturbances, nystagmus

INTERACTIONS: CNS depressants: potentiate effects

PREPARATIONS: Tablet, capsule, syrup

SPECIAL: Many patients are on combination therapy

COMMON EXAMPLES:

Celontin	Milontin
Depakene	Mogadon
Dilantin	Mysoline
Epival	Rivotril
Mebaral	Tegretol
Mebroin	Zarontin
Mesantoin	

TYPE(S): **Monoamine Oxidase (MAOIs) (psychotropics)**

ACTIONS: Affects mood & behavior:
1. Blocks impulse transmission @ the synapse
2. Inhibits catecholamine breakdown

Note: Very long duration.

USES:
1. Moderate-severe depression (usually refractory to TCAs)
2. Atypical depression & phobic disorders (drug of choice)
3. Prevention of "panic attacks"
4. Depressive disorders (atypical, neurotic, reactive)

ADVERSE EFFECTS:

CVS
- □ **Tachycardia,** PVCs, VT
- □ **Hypotension, sweating**

CNS
- □ **Respiratory depression,** CNS depression, **dizziness,** headache, **irritability,** anxiety, paresthesia, tremor, **seizure, coma**
- □ **Ataxia, fever,** insomnia

Other
- □ N/v, urine retention, constipation
- □ Stiff neck, dry mouth

INTERACTIONS:
1. Antihypertensives: may potentiate effects
2. Sympathomimetics or tyramine-rich foods & drinks: may potentiate effects (may induce hypertensive crisis)
3. CNS depressants: may potentiate effects

PREPARATIONS: Tablet

SPECIAL: OD effects may persist for days

COMMON EXAMPLES:
Marplan
Nardil
Parnate

TYPE(S): **Tricyclics (TCAs) (psychotropics)**

ACTIONS: Mechanism of action is not exactly clear:

1. Antidepressant effects
2. Mild sedative effects
3. Cholinergic blockade → anticholinergic effects
4. May inhibit catecholamine breakdown
5. Peripheral α-blockade → anti-α effects
6. Impairs cardiac depolarization & conduction
7. (−) inotropy

Note: Very long duration (may persist for days).

USES:

1. Severe endogenous depression (drug of choice)
2. Prevention of "panic attacks"

ADVERSE EFFECTS:

CVS
- Orthostatic **hypotension,** bradycardia
- (Wide complex) **tachycardia, arrhythmia, PVCs, conduction defects** (widened QRS, prolonged PR & QT, ST & T-wave abnormalities, AV blocks)
- May precipitate CHF

CNS
- *Initially:* confusion, anxiety, sweating, ataxia, vomiting
- May precipitate mania & psychosis
- *Later:* CNS depression, delirium, hallucinations, coma, muscle rigidity, seizure, respiratory depression, apnea

Other
- Anticholinergic effects (fever; hot, flushed skin; dry mucous membranes; pupil dilation; urine retention)
- Anti-α effects (hypotension, sedation, cardiac depression)

INTERACTIONS:

1. Sympathomimetics: may potentiate effects
2. CNS depressants: may potentiate effects

PREPARATIONS: Tablet, capsule

SPECIAL:

1. Ingestion of 1-2 g is potentially lethal
2. Physostigmine (Antilirium), a cholinergic, may reverse some cholinergic adverse effects
3. Clinically related to phenothiazines
4. OD effects may persist for days

COMMON EXAMPLES:

Adapin	Norpramin
Anafranil	Pamelor
Asendin	Pertofrane
Aventyl	Sinequan
Desyrel	Surmontil
Elavil	Tofranil
Etrafon	Triadapin
Limbitrol	Triptil
Ludiomil	Vivactil

TYPE(S): **Insulin (Pancreatic Hormone)**

ACTIONS:
1. Facilitates glucose transmembrane transport & stimulates carbohydrate metabolism
2. Facilitates glucose storage (as glycogen), primarily in the liver, muscle, & kidney

Note: Insulin preparations differ primarily in onset, peak, & duration of action which may vary slightly between manufacturers.

Insulin type	Time (hr)		
	Onset	Peak	Duration
Short Acting			
Regular (Toronto)	0.5-1	2.5-5	5-8
Semilente	1-1.5	5-10	12-16
Intermediate Acting			
NPH	1.5-2	4-12	24-48
Lente	2-2.5	7-15	22-48
Long Acting			
PZI	4-7	10-30	36+
Ultralente	4-7	8-30	28-36+

USES: Diabetes that cannot be controlled by diet alone:
1. Diabetics who cannot produce or excrete adequate amounts of insulin: usually type I (IDDM or juvenile) diabetics
2. In place of oral hypoglycemic therapy in patients with complications

ADVERSE EFFECTS: Other
- □ **Hypoglycemia**
- □ Hypokalemia, electrolyte depletion

INTERACTIONS:

1. ETOH, β-blockers, MAOIs, anabolic steroids, salicylates: may potentiate hypoglycemic effects
2. Corticosteroids, thiazides, catecholamines: may diminish hypoglycemic effects

PREPARATIONS:

Multidose vial, penfill (SC or IM injection)
Some are combination products

SPECIAL:

1. "Epi" may reverse hypoglycemic effects
2. May be on a combination of different insulin preparations
3. Extracted from beef or pork pancreas or produced from genetic engineering

> **Note:** Insulin is a protein & is destroyed in the GI tract. It must be given parenterally. The abdomen, thigh, & arm are common sites.

COMMON EXAMPLES:

Humilin	Novolin
Iletin	Velosulin

TYPE(S):		**Oral Hypoglycemics (sulfonylureas)**
ACTIONS:		Stimulates pancreatic beta cells to produce & secrete insulin

> **Note:** Oral Hypoglycemics differ primarily in onset, peak, & duration of action

USES:		To control hyperglycemia in patients whose diabetes cannot be controlled by diet alone & when Insulin therapy is inappropriate: usually type II (NIDDM or adult) diabetics
ADVERSE EFFECTS:	**Other**	□ **Severe & prolonged hypoglycemia** (especially when accompanied by acute ETOH OD) □ Possible associated hypoglycemic seizure

> **Note:** Hypoglycemia may persist despite IV Dextrose or may recur (since oral hypoglycemics are longer lasting than Dextrose).

INTERACTIONS:

1. ETOH, anabolic steroids, MAOIs, oral anticoagulants, salicylates, sulfonamides, β-blockers: may potentiate hypoglycemic effects
2. Corticosteroids, glucagon, thiazides, catecholamines: may diminish hypoglycemic effects

PREPARATIONS: Tablet

SPECIAL: Provides an alternative to IV insulin

COMMON EXAMPLES:

Diaβeta	Euglucon
Diabinese	Mobenol
Dimelor	Orinase

Antihypertensives[105]

TYPE(S):		**Various (Vasodilators, Sympatholytics, β-blockers, Diuretics, & combination products)**
ACTIONS:		Various mechanisms: 1. Vasodilation (→ decreased BP) 2. ACE inhibitors (→ reduced vasoconstriction) 3. Sympatholytics (→ reduced vessel tone) 4. α-blockade (→ reduced SVR) 5. Diuresis (→ decreased volume)
USES:		1. Hypertension, CHF 2. Na^+ retention, edema, ascites
ADVERSE EFFECTS:	**CVS**	□ Orthostatic to profound **hypotension, syncope,** flushing □ Rebound hypertension, reflex tachycardia, arrhythmia, **angina,** PVCs
	CNS	□ Drowsiness, **dizziness,** confusion, sedation, **headache**
	Other	□ Fluid & Na^+ retention → CHF, electrolyte imbalance □ N/v/d, abdominal pain, muscle cramps
INTERACTIONS:		MAOIs: may potentiate hypotensive effects
PREPARATIONS:		Tablet, capsule
SPECIAL:		Some are combination products
COMMON EXAMPLES:		Aldomet, Capoten, Catapres, Combipres, Loniten, Minipress, Serpasil, Viskazide

[105]There are many different types of antihypertensives. Specific information is beyond the scope of this pocket reference.

TYPE(S): **Primarily Phenothiazines (major tranquilizers) (psychotropics)**

ACTIONS:
1. Phenothiazines alter behavior in such a way as to enable the patient to cope with illness and function in daily activities without excessive sedation.
2. Some also have antiemetic or anticholinergic effects.

> **Note:** Tranquilizers induce calmness & sedation without excessively depressing LOC.

USES:
1. Acute & chronic control of behavioral disorders resulting from mental illness:
   a. Schizophrenia, recurrent mania
   b. Psychotic disorders
   c. Anxiety disorders
   d. Behavioral disorders
2. Prevention of n/v

ADVERSE EFFECTS:

CVS
- □ Hypotension, bradycardia, arrhythmia, AV blocks

CNS
- □ Respiratory depression, **CNS depression, sedation, drowsiness,** confusion, dizziness, weakness, tremor, seizure, coma

Other
- □ Extrapyramidal effects (primarily muscle spasms)
- □ Anticholinergic effects (dry mouth, nasal congestion, blurred vision, salivation)

INTERACTIONS:
1. Opiates, barbiturates, ETOH, & other CNS depressants: may potentiate effects
2. "Epi": may be ineffective in reversing hypotension (may in fact potentiate the hypotension)

PREPARATIONS: Tablet, solution, suspension, syrup, suppository

SPECIAL:
1. Diphenhydramine (Benadryl) or Benztropine (Cogentin) may counteract some adverse effects

COMMON EXAMPLES:

Haldol	Peridol	Sparine
Haloperidol	Permitil	Stelazine
Mellaril	Quide	Trilafon
Nozinan	Serentil	

Beta-Blockers

TYPE(S): **Sympathetic Blocker**

ACTIONS: Some selectively block β_1 (cardioselective) or β_2 (bronchoselective) receptors; some are nonselective.

> **Note:** Selective β-blockers are usually dose dependent (tend to lose β_2 selectivity in higher doses)

USES:
1. Mild-moderate hypertension
2. Prevention of recurrent angina
3. Prevention of recurring tachyarrhythmias
4. Migraines

ADVERSE EFFECTS:

CVS
- □ May precipitate or aggravate COPD, asthma, **bronchospasm,** & increased airway resistance
- □ **Hypotension, bradycardia,** AV block, **CHF**

CNS
- □ Fatigue, headache, hallucinations, seizure, coma

Other
- □ N/v, may induce **hypoglycemia**

INTERACTIONS:
1. Sympathomimetics: block β-effects (patient may be unable to mount a tachycardic response to hypovolemia)
2. Ca^{++} blockers: potentiate bradycardia & myocardial depression
3. Cardiac glycosides: potentiate bradycardia
4. "Epi": severe vasoconstriction
5. Diuretics: may potentiate antihypertensive effects

PREPARATIONS: Tablet

SPECIAL:
1. Acute withdrawal may precipitate angina (due to increased sensitivity to catecholamines)
2. Often used in combination therapy

COMMON EXAMPLES:

Betaloc	Lopressor
Blocadren	Sotacor
Corgard	Tenormin
Inderal	Visken

TYPE(S): **Sympathomimetics**

ACTIONS: Most are β_2 selective (some are not)

1. Bronchodilation (via β_2 stimulation)
2. Some β_1 effects
3. Little or no α-stimulation

> **Note:** Some are catecholamines; some are not. They differ primarily in their onset & duration

USES: Prevention/Tx of bronchospasm caused by reversible obstructive airway disease (COPD → asthma, bronchitis, emphysema)

ADVERSE EFFECTS:

CVS
- □ Excessive cardiac stimulation, tachycardia, palpitation, hypertension
- □ May precipitate angina, AMI, PVCs, arrhythmia
- □ Possible hypotension, sweating

CNS
- □ Excessive CNS stimulation (anxiety to seizure)
- □ Headache, dizziness, drowsiness, weakness, fatigue
- □ Paresthesia

Other
- □ N/v, heartburn, bad taste, muscle cramps, dry nose & throat
- □ May cause severe paradoxical bronchospasm from repeated excessive use

INTERACTIONS:

1. β-blockers: may block effects
2. MAOIs, TCAs: may potentiate effects

PREPARATIONS: Aerosol, tablet, suppository, nebulizer solution

SPECIAL:

1. Aerosolized drugs may not reach the smaller airways, especially in the presence of bronchospasm & thick mucous plugs (the nebulizer solution will be much more effective)
2. Aerosol sympathomimetics have the potential for patient tolerance & abuse
3. These patients may also be on steroids & antibiotics
4. Some are combination products
5. OD effects may be reversed by a β-blocker such as Propranolol (Inderal)

COMMON EXAMPLES:

Alupent	Bronkaid
Berotec	Bronkometer
Brethaire	Bronkosol
Brethine	Vaponefrin
Bricanyl	Ventolin

TYPE(S): **Theophyllines**

ACTIONS:
1. Bronchodilation & vasodilation
2. Respiratory stimulation
3. Diuresis
4. (+) chronotropy, (+) inotropy

USES: Prevention/Tx of bronchospasm caused by reversible obstructive airway disease (COPD → asthma, bronchitis, emphysema) & related bronchospastic disorders

ADVERSE EFFECTS:

CVS
- **Hypotension,** angina, **tachycardia, palpitation,** arrhythmia, **PVCs,** flushing

CNS
- Headache, nervousness, irritability, **anxiety,** excitement, **dizziness,** mild delirium, insomnia, fever, tremor, **seizure,** coma
- Increased respiratory rate

Other
- N/v/d, anorexia, abdominal cramps, hematemesis
- Diuresis, dehydration
- Visual or auditory disturbances

INTERACTIONS:
1. β-blockers: may oppose effects
2. Barbiturates, Phenytoin: may decrease Theophylline blood levels

PREPARATIONS: Tablet, aerosol, elixir, syrup, suppository

SPECIAL:
1. Children are very sensitive: toxic to therapeutic ratio is small
2. Some are combination products

COMMON EXAMPLES:

Choledyl	Somophyllin
Phyllocontin	Tedral
Quibron	Theo-Dur

Calcium Channel Blockers[106]

TYPE(S): **Antiarrhythmic, Antihypertensive, Antianginal**

ACTIONS: Blocks entry of Ca^{++} into the cell (especially cardiac & vascular smooth muscle) →:

1. (−) chronotropy
2. (−) inotropy
3. (−) dromotropy
4. Vasodilation (including coronary)
5. Bronchodilation
6. Inhibits coronary artery spasm

> **Note:** Verapamil's most potent activity is electrophysiologic.
> Nifedipine's most potent activity is hemodynamic.
> Diltiazem acts like a less potent combination of the two.

USES:

Nifedipine, Verapamil, & Diltiazem:

1. Angina from coronary artery spasm
2. Chronic stable angina (effort associated)

Verapamil:
PSVT, A-fib, A-flutter

ADVERSE EFFECTS

Diltiazem:

CVS □ Conduction disturbances, **arrhythmia,** hypotension, bradycardia, CHF; flushing, **peripheral edema**

CNS □ **Headache, fatigue, drowsiness,** dizziness, nervousness, CNS depression, confusion, insomnia

Other □ N/v/d, **rash**

Verapamil & Nifedipine: See drug pages

INTERACTIONS:

1. "Dig": may increase "Dig" blood levels
2. β-blockers: may potentiate some effects → heart failure

---

[106]Diltiazem, Nifedipine, & Verapamil are the most common Ca^{++} blockers in current use. Specific information is beyond the scope of this pocket reference.

PREPARATIONS: Tablet, capsule (PO, SL)

SPECIAL: Often used in combination therapy

COMMON EXAMPLES:
Adalat
Cardizem
Isoptin

(Cardiotonics) Cardiac Glycosides

TYPE(S): **Digitalis ("Dig") Preparations**

ACTIONS: Promotes movement of Ca^{++} into the cell.

1. (+) inotrope
2. (−) chronotrope
3. (−) dromotrope
4. Improves atrial conduction

> **Note:** "Dig" glycosides vary in potency, onset, & duration of action. They are generally long-acting.

USES:

1. CHF, post-MI
2. A-fib, A-flutter
3. SVTs

ADVERSE EFFECTS:

CVS
- **May exacerbate CHF, almost any arrhythmia or conduction defect** (usually conduction disturbances, PACs, PVCs, SVTs)
- Hypotension

CNS
- **Fatigue, weakness, agitation, hallucinations,** behavioral changes, headache, dizziness, vertigo, confusion, **anxiety,** paresthesia, insomnia

Other
- N/v/d, anorexia, malaise
- **Visual disturbances**
- Hypokalemia

INTERACTIONS: Diuretics, Ca^{++}, Quinidine, Amiodarone, Ca^{++} blockers, catecholamines: may precipitate "Dig" toxicity

PREPARATIONS: Tablet, capsule

SPECIAL:

1. Toxicity is more frequent in patients with hypokalemia, hypocalcemia, or hypomagnesemia
2. About 7%-40% of patients on "Dig" develop some symptoms of toxicity
3. Digitalized patients may develop more serious & resistant arrhythmias following cardioversion. Use of very low energy levels & prophylactic Lidocaine or Phenytoin may prevent this

COMMON EXAMPLES:

Cedilanid
Crystodigin
Digitaline
Lanoxin
Novodigoxin

Diuretics[107]

TYPE(S): **Various (primarily Thiazides, Loop, & combination products with Antihypertensives, β-blockers, & Aldosterone antagonists)**

ACTIONS:
1. Diuresis
2. Promotes Na^+ excretion
3. Vasodilation

USES:
1. Hypertension
2. Chronic fluid overload (CHF, pulmonary, peripheral edema)
3. Liver cirrhosis with ascites & edema
4. Decreased renal function (impairment)
5. Edema (drug induced or from renal origin)

ADVERSE EFFECTS:

CVS
- **Hypovolemia, hypotension, tachycardia,** arrhythmia

CNS
- Drowsiness, **confusion, delirium, dizziness, weakness,** seizure, coma

Other
- **Dehydration, electrolyte imbalance** (most commonly K^+), hyperosmolality, **dry mouth/thirst,** cramps
- May inhibit insulin release → hyperglycemia
- N/v/d
- **Visual or auditory disturbances**

INTERACTIONS: Antihypertensives: increased antihypertensive effects

PREPARATIONS: Tablet, capsule, suppository

SPECIAL:
1. Also known as "water pills"
2. These patients are often on K^+ supplements
3. ECG may show prominent P-waves, diminished T-waves, & presence of U-waves

COMMON EXAMPLES:

Aldactazide	Dyazide
Aldactone	Lasix
Duretic	Moduret

[107]There are many different types of diuretics. Specific information is beyond the scope of this pocketbook.

Sedative-Hypnotics

TYPE(S): **Primarily Barbiturates, Benzodiazepines**
Also Piperidines, Carbamates

ACTIONS: Sedatives induce CNS depression, sedation, & "calm the nerves"
Hypnotics induce & maintain sleep

> **Note:** Duration of action varies with each drug. Some may be extremely long.

USES: Some are for daytime use, some are for nighttime use.

1. Anxiety, tension, stress, apprehension, irritability, excitement, insomnia
2. Chronic behavioral disorders
3. Psychotherapy
4. Seizure disorders

ADVERSE EFFECTS:

CVS
- □ **Hypotension,** pulmonary edema

CNS
- □ **CNS or respiratory depression, drowsiness, dizziness, weakness,** confusion, delirium, headache, **ataxia,** slurred speech, hypnosis (Paradoxical excitement in the elderly)
- □ Possible paresthesia, seizure, coma
- □ Nightmares, **hangover**

Other
- □ Extrapyramidal reactions
- □ Anticholinergic effects[108]
- □ Parkinson-like reactions (especially in children)
- □ N/v/d, rash
- □ Withdrawal syndrome[109]

INTERACTIONS:

1. ETOH, other CNS depressants: excessive CNS & respiratory depression
2. MAOIs: inhibit barbiturate metabolism

PREPARATIONS: Tablet, capsule, suppository

---

[108]Dry mouth; hot, dry red skin; blurred vision; urine retention.
[109]Anxiety, tachycardia, CNS effects.

SPECIAL:

1. Some have potential for tolerance, abuse, & addiction from chronic use
2. Some are combination products

COMMON EXAMPLES:

Amytal	Nembutal
Butisol	Nodular
Dalmane	Placidyl
Day-Barb	Plexonal
Doriden	Restoril
Halcion	Seconal
Mandrax	Tuinal
Mogadon	Tranxene

Section Six

Glossary
Bibliography
Directory

GLOSSARY

Adrenergic (sympathomimetic)- nerve fibers (sympathetic) that release and receptors that respond to catecholamines.

Afterload- amount of left ventricular volume immediately following systole. Primarily dependent on SVR.

Agonist- a drug with high affinity for a receptor and causes activity at the receptor site.

Antagonist- a drug with high affinity for a receptor but prevents or reduces the activity at the receptor site.

Anticholinergic (parasympatholytic)- blocks actions of ACh, thus blocking parasympathetic or other cholinergic nerve fibers (i.e., PNS blockade and potentiation of the SNS).

Automaticity- spontaneous, involuntary ability to generate action potentials.

Blocker- an agent that occupies the receptor site for the drug, preventing its usual effect(s).

Bolus- a concentrated mass of drug (usually given IV push).

Catecholamine(s)- neurohormone(s) (or neurotransmitters) having sympathomimetic action; produced largely by the adrenal medulla and adrenergic nerve endings. They are dopamine, norepinephrine, and epinephrine. Act as neurotransmitters in the CNS.

Cholinergic (parasympathomimetic)- activated or transmitted by ACh. Nerve fibers (parasympathetic) that release and receptors that respond to ACh. Also, any that produce the same type of effect.

Chronotropy- rate of contraction (i.e., heart rate).

Colloid- aggregates of molecules, some of which are proteins (larger than crystalloid molecules but not large enough to settle out under the influence of gravity, & does not pass through cellular membranes) suspended in a liquid medium. Has oncotic pressure and remains within the intravascular space.

Cross-matched- process of comparing donor blood product with recipient blood to determine compatibility.

Crystalloid- a readily soluble substance (usually a salt) that, in solution passes easily through cellular membranes. Has no oncotic pressure. Has osmotic pressure and will diffuse out of the intravascular space within an hour to equilibrate with extracellular fluid. Does not contain proteins (i.e., noncolloid).

Depressant- an agent that reduces the functional activity of the body or any of its organs (by producing muscular relaxation).

Dromotropy- conduction through the AV node.

Endogenous- developing or originating within the organism or arising from causes within the organism.

Exogenous- developing or originating outside the organism or arising from causes outside the organism.

Extrapyramidal- outside the pyramidal tract. Spasmodic movements, muscle spasms, loss of fine motor function.

Extravasation- a discharge or escape from a vessel into the tissues. May cause severe burning, cellulitis, or phlebitis and lead to tissue necrosis.

Generic name- the nonproprietary or chemical name.

Group (type) specific- refers to a blood product of the same ABO group as the patient.

Half-life- the time required for drug concentration in plasma or total body to be reduced by one-half.

Hypersensitivity- a state of altered reactivity producing an exaggerated response to a foreign agent (allergic response). Reacts with characteristic symptoms.

Infiltration- refers to an IV solution that has been infused into tissue rather than a vessel. Characterized by a decreased IV flow rate; localized edema; cool, pale, hard area.

Infusion- the therapeutic introduction of a fluid (other than blood) into a vein. Flows in by gravity.

Inotropy- strength and force of muscular contraction (i.e., cardiac output).

Intraosseous- within the bone (e.g., infusion into the medullary sinus).

Irritability- abnormally sensitive to a slight stimuli.

Irritation- action that produces slight or temporary damage to tissues.

Necrosis- tissue death. Usually small localized areas.

Parenteral- not through the alimentary canal but rather by injection (IV, SC, IM, IO).

Peripheral (systemic) vascular resistance- see systemic.

Phlebitis- venous inflammation (usually the inner walls) characterized by tenderness, redness, puffiness, warmth, induration, soreness.

Physiological action- action caused by the drug when given in the concentrations normally present in the body (applies only to drugs that are derived from normal body chemicals).

Potentiation- enhancement of the effect of one drug by another so that the combined effect is greater than the sum of the effects of each one alone.

Preload- amount of left ventricular volume immediately preceding systole. Primarily dependent on venous return. (Also known as left ventricular end diastolic pressure, LVEDP.)

Pressor- an agent which increases SVR and hence increases BP.

Proprietary name- the trade name.

Receptor site (cell)- a specific chemical grouping on the cell surface capable of combining specifically with an antigen. A predictable sequence of responses will occur.

Reconstitute- to mix (usually dissolving a powder with a liquid).

Reentry- a postulated mechanism by which a premature impulse may be coupled to a normal impulse, creating a circuit or "circus effect" and leading to arrhythmias.

Refractory- not readily yielding to treatment, resistant to treatment.

Stimulant- an agent that excites (increases) functional activity of the body or any of its organs.

Synergistic- acting together, enhancing the effect of another agent or force. Joint action(s) of agents such that their combined effect is greater than the algebraic sum of their individual effects.

Systemic vascular resistance- resistance exerted primarily by the arterioles.

Therapeutic action- beneficial action of a drug to correct a body dysfunction. The desired effect of the drug.

Titrate- administer until the desired effect is achieved.

Tolerance- reduced responsiveness after repeated administration of a drug requiring progressively larger doses.

Toxicity- the serum level of a drug that causes the most severe adverse effects (which may be life threatening).

Trade name- the proprietary name.

Transfusion- therapeutic introduction of blood into a vein.

Venous capacitance- ability to "store" blood, i.e., venous pooling. Commonly mediated by smooth muscle relaxation and venodilation as a result of decreased sympathetic stimulation. Increased venous capacitance reduces preload.

BIBLIOGRAPHY

American Association of Blood Banks, *Blood Transfusion Therapy - A Physician's Handbook.* 4th ed., Arlington, Virginia, 1987.

American College of Surgeons, *Advanced Trauma Life Support-Instructor Manual,* 1989.

American Heart Association, *Textbook of Advanced Cardiac Life Support.* Dallas, Texas, 1987.

American Hospital Formulary Service: Drug Information 1987.

Bledsoe, B.E., *Manual of Emergency Drugs.* Fort Worth, Texas, Prentice-Hall, 1984.

Canadian Pharmaceutical Association, *Compendium of Pharmaceuticals And Specialties 1988.* 23rd ed.

Canadian Red Cross Society Blood Services, *Clinical Guide to Transfusion Products & Practices.* 2nd ed., Ottawa, Ontario, 1987.

Caroline, N.L., *Emergency Care in the Streets.* 3rd ed., Little, Brown and Company Inc., Boston, Massachusetts, 1987.

Crowell, R., Jefferis, L., *Paramedic Pharmacology Handbook.* Paramedic Training Institute, Department of Health Services Los Angeles County, California, 3rd Printing, 1982.

Dorland's Illustrated Medical Dictionary. 27th ed., Saunders, 1988.

Drugs of Choice from the Medical Letter. The Medical Letter Inc., New York, New York, 1985.

Emergency, Drug Watch Articles '85-'88. Hare Publications, California.

Gazzaniga, A.B. et al., *Emergency Care Principles & Practices for the EMT-Paramedic.* 2nd ed., Prentice-Hall, California, 1982.

Govoni, L.E., Hayes, J.D., *Drugs and Nursing Implications.* 5th ed., Appleton-Century-Crofts, Connecticut, 1985.

Grauer K., Cavallaro, D.L., *ACLS: Certification Preparation & A Comprehensive Review.* 2nd ed., C.V. Mosby Co., 1987.

Greenway, K.T., Jarvis, D.A., *Pediatric Advanced Life Support.* 2nd ed., Hamilton, Ontario, 1987.

Jenson, S.A., *Paramedic Handbook.* Denver, Colorado, Multi-Media Inc., 1983.

Khan, G.M., *Manual of Cardiac Drug Therapy.* Ottawa, Ontario, Bailliere Tindall, 1985.

Knoben, J.E., Anderson P.O., *Handbook of Clinical Drug Data.* 5th ed., Drug Intelligence Publications, Inc., 1986.

Lock, G.R., *Common Drugs Given by Paramedics.* Nanton, Alberta, 1985.

Nursing 87 Drug Handbook. Springhouse Corporation, 1987.

Walraven, G. et al., *Handbook Of Emergency Drugs.* San Diego, California, R.J. Brady Co., 1978.

DIRECTORY

NUMBERS

Dispatch

Base

Hospitals

Poison Control

Police

Fire

Hazardous Materials

Search & Rescue

Coast Guard

Miscellaneous

FREQUENCIES

International Distress	121.500
Aviation Emergency Medical	129.275

Mayday → Distress **Pan Pan → Urgency** **Security → Safety**

Index

C

D

M

N

O

P